WHO EXPERT CONSULTATION ON RABIES

First report

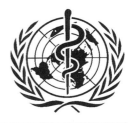

World Health Organization
Geneva 2005

WHO Library Cataloguing-in-Publication Data

WHO Expert Consultation on Rabies (2004 : Geneva, Switzerland)
   WHO Expert Consultation on Rabies : first report.

   (WHO technical report series ; 931)

   1.Rabies — prevention and control   2.Rabies vaccines   3.Rabies virus
   4.Epidemiologic surveillance   5.Guidelines   I.Title   II.Series.

   ISBN 92 4 120931 3   (NLM classification: WC 550)
   ISSN 0512-3054

© World Health Organization 2005

The designations employed and the presentation of the material in this publication do not imply the expression of any opinion whatsoever on the part of the World Health Organization concerning the legal status of any country, territory, city or area or of its authorities, or concerning the delimitation of its frontiers or boundaries. Dotted lines on maps represent approximate border lines for which there may not yet be full agreement.

The mention of specific companies or of certain manufacturers' products does not imply that they are endorsed or recommended by the World Health Organization in preference to others of a similar nature that are not mentioned. Errors and omissions excepted, the names of proprietary products are distinguished by initial capital letters.

All reasonable precautions have been taken by the World Health Organization to verify the information contained in this publication. However, the published material is being distributed without warranty of any kind, either express or implied. The responsibility for the interpretation and use of the material lies with the reader. In no event shall the World Health Organization be liable for damages arising from its use.

This publication contains the collective views of an international group of experts and does not necessarily represent the decisions or the stated policy of the World Health Organization.

This publication contains information on certain vaccines that international experts appointed by WHO have found to be safe and efficacious when applied by the intradermal route for rabies pre- and post-exposure prophylaxis.

The evaluation of safety and efficacy is based on the assessment of a review of published articles (in peer-reviewed journals) on clinical studies (on safety, immunogenicity and efficacy) conducted with these products and an analysis of laboratory tests results carried out as part of these studies by independent laboratories or for the control of these products by national control authorities and/or by the manufacturers. Therefore, inclusion in this publication does not constitute a warranty of the suitability of any individual batch of vaccine for a particular purpose. The responsibility for the quality, safety and efficacy of each individual batch of vaccines remains with the manufacturer.

Furthermore, WHO does not warrant that:

1. the vaccines that have been found to be safe and efficacious by the intradermal route will continue to be so;

2. the vaccines have obtained regulatory approval for post-exposure prophylaxis of rabies (or any other disease) in every country of the world, or that their use is otherwise in accordance with the national laws and regulations of any country, including but not limited to patents laws.

In addition, WHO wishes to alert procuring United Nations agencies that the improper storage, handling and transportation of vaccines may affect their quality, efficacy and safety. WHO disclaims any and all liability and responsibility for any injury, death, loss, damage or other prejudice of any kind whatsoever that may arise as a result of or in connection with the procurement, distribution and use of any vaccine or other product mentioned in this publication.

The information in this publication should not be used for promotional purposes.

Typeset in Hong Kong
Printed in Singapore

Contents

WHO Expert Consultation on Rabies

Geneva, 5–8 October 2004

Participants

Dr D. Briggs, Adjunct Professor, Department of Diagnostic Medicine/Pathobiology, College of Veterinary Medicine, Kansas State University, Manhattan, KS, USA

Dr H. Bourhy, Head, Rabies Unit, Department of Ecosystems and Epidemiology of Infectious Diseases, Pasteur Institute and Director, WHO Collaborating Centre for Reference and Research on Rabies, Paris, France

Dr S. Cleaveland, Senior Lecturer, Tropical Animal Health, Centre for Tropical Veterinary Medicine, University of Edinburgh, Easter Bush Veterinary Centre, Roslin, Midlothian, Scotland

Dr F. Cliquet, Director, Research Laboratory for Rabies and Pathology of Wild Animals and Director, WHO Collaborating Centre for Research and Management on Zoonoses Control, National Centre on Veterinary and Food Studies (AFSSA), Malzéville, France

Dr H. Ertl, Professor and Programme Leader, Immunology Programme, The Wistar Institute and Director, WHO Collaborating Centre for Reference and Research on Rabies, Philadelphia, PA, USA

Dr A. Fayaz, Head, Virology Department, Pasteur Institute of Iran and Director, WHO Collaborating Centre for Reference and Research on Rabies, Tehran, Islamic Republic of Iran

Dr A. Fooks, Head, Veterinary Laboratories Agency, Department of Virology and Director, WHO Collaborating Centre for the Characterization of Rabies and Rabies-related Viruses, Addlestone, Weybridge, England

Dr T. Hemachudha, Professor of Medicine and Neurology, Chulalongkorn University Hospital, Bangkok, Thailand

Dr R.L. Ichhpujani, Deputy Director General, Directorate General of Health Services, Ministry of Health and Family Welfare, New Delhi, India

Dr W. R. Kaboyo, Assistant Commissioner for Veterinary Public Health and Zoonoses Control, Ministry of Health, Kampala, Uganda (*Rapporteur*)

Dr H. Koprowski, Professor, Department of Immunology and Microbiology, Thomas Jefferson University and Director, WHO Collaborating Centre for Neurovirology, Philadelphia, PA, USA

Dr S. N. Madhusudana, Additional Professor, Department of Neurovirology, National Institute of Mental Health and Neurosciences and Director, WHO Collaborating Centre for Reference and Research in Rabies, Bangalore, India

Dr T. Müller, Senior Scientist and Principal Investigator, Institute of Epidemiology, Federal Research Institute for Animal Virus Diseases and Director, WHO Collaborating Centre for Rabies Surveillance and Research, Wusterhausen, Germany

Dr L. Nel, Professor, Department of Microbiology, University of Pretoria, Faculty of Natural and Agricultural Sciences, Pretoria, South Africa

Dr B. Quiambao, Chief, Clinical Research Division, Research Institute for Tropical Medicine, Metro Manila, Philippines (*Rapporteur*)

Dr C.E. Rupprecht, Head, Rabies Section, Division of Viral and Rickettsial Diseases, Viral and Rickettsial Zoonoses Branch, National Center for Infectious Diseases, Centers for Disease Control and Prevention and Director, WHO Collaborating Centre for Reference and Research on Rabies, Atlanta, GA, USA

Dr N. Salahuddin, President, Infectious Disease Society of Pakistan, Liaquat National Hospital, Karachi, Pakistan

Professor M.K. Sudarshan, Head, Department of Community Medicine, Kempegowda Institute of Medical Sciences, Bangalore, India

Dr N. Tordo, Head, Antiviral Strategies Unit, Department of Virology, Pasteur Institute, Paris, France

Dr A.I. Wandeler, Head, Centre of Expertise for Rabies, Ottawa Laboratory Fallowfield, Canadian Food Inspection Agency and Director, WHO Collaborating Centre for Control, Pathogenesis and Epidemiology of Rabies in Carnivores, Nepean, Ontario, Canada (*Chairman*)

Dr H. Wilde, Professor of Medicine, Department of Medicine, Chulangkorn University, and Senior Consultant Physician, Queen Saovabha Memorial Institute, Thai Red Cross Society, Bangkok, Thailand

Representatives of other organizations[1]

World Organisation for Animal Health (OIE)
Dr F. Cliquet, Director, Research Laboratory for Rabies and Pathology of Wild Animals and Head, OIE Reference Laboratory on Rabies, National Centre on Veterinary and Food Studies (AFSSA), Malzéville, France

Marwar Animal Protection Trust
Mr F. Spinola, Chairman, Marwar Trust, Geneva, Switzerland

Secretariat[2]

Dr A. Belotto, Chief, Veterinary Public Health Unit, Pan American Health Organization/WHO Regional Office for the Americas, Washington, DC, USA

Dr R. Bhatia, Focal Point for Zoonoses, Blood Safety and Clinical Technology, Communicable Diseases, WHO Regional Office for South-East Asia, New Delhi, India

Dr H. Endo, Director, Control, Prevention and Eradication, Communicable Diseases, WHO, Geneva, Switzerland

Dr B. Ganter, Regional Adviser, Communicable Disease Surveillance and Response, Communicable Diseases, WHO Regional Office for Europe, Copenhagen, Denmark

Dr R. Gibert, Scientist, Viral Vaccine Control and Viral Safety Unit, French Agency for Health Product Safety (AFSSAPS), Lyon, France (*Temporary Adviser*)

---

[1] The following representatives were invited, but were unable to attend: Dr J. Domenech, Chief, Animal Health Unit, Animal Health and Production Division, Food and Agriculture Organization of the United Nations (FAO), Rome Italy; and Dr R. Butcher, Consultant, World Society for the Protection of Animals (WSPA), London, England.
[2] Dr R. Ben-Ismaïl, Regional Adviser, Tropical Diseases and Zoonoses/Communicable Disease Control, WHO Regional Office for the Eastern Mediterranean, Cairo, Egypt, was invited, but was unable to attend.

Dr V. Grachev, Deputy Director, Institute of Poliomyelitis and Viral Encephalitides, Academy of Medical Sciences of the Russian Federation, Moscow, Russian Federation (*Temporary Adviser*)

Dr I. Knezevic, Scientist, Quality Assurance and Safety: Biologicals, Immunization, Vaccines and Biologicals, Family and Community Health, WHO, Geneva, Switzerland

Dr D. Mc Adams, Grand Saconnex, Geneva, Switzerland (*Consultant*)

Dr F.-X. Meslin, Coordinator, Strategy Development and Monitoring of Zoonoses, Foodborne Diseases and Kinetoplastidae, Control, Prevention and Eradication, Communicable Diseases, WHO, Geneva, Switzerland (*Secretary*)

Dr E. Miranda, Focal Point for Rabies, Communicable Disease Surveillance and Response, Combating Communicable Diseases, WHO Regional Office for the Western Pacific, Manila, Philippines

Dr Sylvie Morgeaux, Head, Viral Vaccine Control and Viral Safety Unit, French Agency for Health Product Safety (AFSSAPS), Lyon, France (*Temporary Adviser*)

Dr J.-B. Roungou, Regional Adviser on Tropical Diseases, Other Tropical Diseases, Prevention and Control of Communicable Diseases, WHO Regional Office for Africa, Harare, Zimbabwe

1. Introduction

The WHO Expert Consultation on Rabies met in Geneva from 5 to 8 October 2004. Dr Hiroyoshi Endo, Director, Control, Prevention and Eradication, Communicable Diseases welcomed the participants on behalf of the Director-General. He pointed out that more than 99% of all human rabies deaths occur in the developing world, and that the disease has not been brought under control throughout most of the affected countries. Although effective and economical control measures are available, their application in developing countries is hampered by a range of economic, social and political factors.

A major factor in the low level of political commitment to rabies control is a lack of accurate data on the true public health impact of the disease. It is widely recognized that the number of deaths officially reported in most developing countries greatly underestimates the true incidence of disease, with several factors contributing to widespread underreporting. In turn, underreporting leads to lack of attention by national authorities in much of Africa and Asia, and by the international organizations concerned. Disparities in the affordability and accessibility of post-exposure prophylaxis, levels of rabies awareness and risks of exposure to rabid dogs result in a skewed distribution of the disease burden across society, with the major impact falling on members, particularly children, of poor rural communities.

Dr François-Xavier Meslin, Coordinator, Strategy Development and Monitoring of Zoonoses, Foodborne Diseases and Kinetoplastidae reminded the participants of the numerous rabies activities conducted by WHO since the last meeting of WHO Expert Committee on Rabies held in 1991. WHO has been working with its collaborating centres, its rabies specialists and other partners in both the public and private sectors to conduct new assessments of the rabies burden in selected countries as well as globally, to promote the development of alternative technologies, such as the intradermal route for post-exposure prophylaxis, monoclonal antibody cocktail as a replacement for human and equine rabies immunoglobulins and oral vaccination of dogs through vaccine-loaded baits. As part of the new thrust for rabies control in Asia, formulated during the WHO International Consultation on Rabies Control and Eradication in Asia, held in Geneva, Switzerland, in 2001, WHO has convened a number of coordinating meetings in Asia to strengthen national capacity to tackle rabies, raise the level of awareness and develop an inter-regional network of opinion leaders who could bring rabies prevention and control to the forefront.

Dr Alexander Wandeler was elected Chairperson and Dr Betty Quiambao and Dr Winyi Kaboyo were elected Rapporteurs.

The information in this report should be considered the most current information on rabies prevention and control and supersedes that of the eighth report of the WHO Expert Committee on Rabies (1).

1.1 Methods to estimate the burden of rabies

The recognized poor quality of rabies reporting from developing countries has recently prompted several investigations into the distribution of mortality attributable to rabies. In one study, a predictive approach similar to that developed for other contagious diseases was used to estimate human rabies deaths in the United Republic of Tanzania (2). This study used a probability decision-tree method to determine the likelihood of clinical rabies developing in a person following the bite of a suspect rabid dog. In addition, in 2003 a WHO working group was established to estimate the global burden of rabies (3). This working group defined modalities for the reassessment of the public health and economic burden of rabies in Africa and Asia by applying data derived from these regions to the probability decision tree model, and thereby presenting a data-driven assessment of the human and economic costs of rabies in the developing world. In addition, a disability-adjusted life year (DALY) score for rabies was calculated and compared with those of other infectious diseases. Furthermore WHO requested the Association for the Prevention and Control of Rabies in India to conduct a multicentre study to assess the current burden of rabies in India (4). For the WHO European Region and the Region of the Americas, data on the economic burden were collected from the literature.

1.2 Estimated burden of rabies in the world

The highest financial expenditure in any country is the cost of rabies post-exposure prophylaxis. The type of vaccine, vaccine regimen and route of administration as well as the type of immunoglobulin used all significantly influence the cost of treatment. In addition to the expense of rabies biologicals are expenditures for the physician, hospital, the loss of income as a result of the need to physically visit a clinic (or to accompany someone else to a clinic), and the emotional and psychological impact of post-exposure prophylaxis.

The use of nerve-tissue vaccines is still widespread because of its assumed low production cost. However, these vaccines are responsible for severe and long-term side-effects in an estimated 0.3 to 0.8 per 1000 cases. The overall cost of these side-effects has not been evaluated, because of the poor reporting rate in the countries where these treatments are still being used. However, the duration of the incurred disability can be from 4.9 months (on average for a Semple vaccine) to 6.6 months (for a suckling-mouse brain vaccine), leading to considerable loss of income. Costs of rabies prevention, control and elimination in animal reservoirs and losses in the animal production sector in particular must also be taken into account.

Africa and Asia. Human mortality from endemic canine rabies was estimated to be 55 000 deaths per year (90% CI: 24 500–90 800) with 56% of the deaths estimated to occur in Asia and 44% in Africa. The majority (84%) of these deaths occur in rural areas. Deaths caused by rabies are responsible for 1.74 (90% CI: 0.25–4.57) million DALYs lost each year. An additional 0.04 million DALYs are lost annually through morbidity and mortality following side-effects of nerve-tissue vaccines, and the psychological impact of fear and trauma induced by suspect rabid dog bites. The latter is the most difficult to translate into a monetary value, but an estimate has been included into a model translating all these components into indirect DALYs. The psychological burden of rabies amounts to 32 385 DALYs in Africa and 139 893 DALYs in Asia. The estimated annual cost of rabies in Africa and Asia is US$ 583.5 (90% CI: 540–626) million, with most of this cost being borne by Asian countries where large amounts of post-exposure prophylaxis are administered (Asia: US$ 563 (90% CI: 520–605.8) million, Africa: US$ 20.5 (90% CI: 19.3–21.8) million). The majority of all post-exposure prophylaxis expenditures are borne by patients who can least afford to pay. For example, in India, patients pay for nearly half of the financial burden attributed to rabies (data summarized from a study carried out by the Association for the Prevention and Control of Rabies in India) (*4*). In Africa and Asia, the annual cost of livestock losses as a result of rabies is estimated to be US$ 12.3 million.

United States of America. The estimated total annual expenditure for rabies prevention amounts to US$ 300 million in the USA (source: United States Centers for Disease Control and Prevention). Several states are attempting to eliminate raccoon rabies in the hope of decreasing the growing need for post-exposure prophylaxis that has followed an ever expanding rabies epizootic in the raccoon population. The campaigns require permanent surveillance and the maintenance of a costly barrier to maintain the country's rabies-free status.

Europe. The red fox is the predominant reservoir of rabies viruses. In France, the cumulative cost of fox rabies control including oral vaccination during the period 1986–1995 was estimated to be US$ 261 million (5).

Latin America. The budget assigned to the national programmes for control of rabies, excluding that of Brazil, was US$ 10 980 892 in 2000 and US$ 22 215 289 in 2001 (6)). Brazil evaluated its own budget for rabies prevention at US$ 28 million in 2004 (S. Garay, personal communication, 2004). These expenses include the cost of vaccines for humans and dogs, immunoglobulins, laboratory diagnosis, medical and veterinary staff, training of staff and dog vaccination campaigns. The costs incurred by people seeking treatment (those related to time lost, loss of income, and side-effects) were not included in these figures, neither was the cost of bat-related rabies in humans or cattle. Vampire bat rabies-related losses are largely underreported. A 1985 estimate brought the death toll in cattle to 100 000 heads per year, at an annual estimated cost of US$ 30 million.

According to the annual per capita gross national income, a full rabies post-exposure prophylaxis course represents as much as 3.87% of the gross national income for a person in Asia and 5.80% for a person in Africa. These figures can rise considerably when more expensive, but safer cell-culture vaccines are used. For example, the cost of post-exposure prophylaxis using a cell-culture vaccine would be equivalent to 51 days' wages for an average African citizen, and 31 days' wages for an average Asian citizen. The total global expenditure for rabies prevention is well over US$ 1 billion annually, but it should be understood that this is a significant underestimate, because of poor surveillance and underreporting in many developing countries, and the absence of coordination between all the players involved. The costs will continue to increase dramatically as more and more countries begin to use modern cell-culture or purified embryonated egg vaccines and as public demand for safe and efficacious treatment increases, which will also, in turn, increase the number of requests for post-exposure prophylaxis. Almost all human deaths caused by rabies worldwide originate from Asia and Africa. Without the use of preventive intervention, i.e. post-exposure prophylaxis, the total number of predicted human rabies deaths in Asia and Africa would be 330 304 (90% CI: 141 844–563 515).

2. Classification of lyssaviruses

2.1 Distinguishing features of lyssaviruses

The etiologic agents of rabies encephalitis belong to the *Mononegavirales* order, *Rhabdoviridae* family and *Lyssavirus* genus.

Lyssaviruses have a 12 kb-long non-segmented RNA genome of negative polarity encoding five viral proteins (3' to 5'): nucleoprotein N, phosphoprotein P, matrix protein M, glycoprotein G and polymerase L. The lyssavirus particle has a bullet-shaped form, 100–300 nm in length and 75 nm in diameter (7). It is composed of two structural and functional units:

(i) the outer envelope covered with spike-like projections (10 nm in length) corresponding to G-protein trimers which recognize specific viral receptors on susceptible cell membranes;
(ii) the internal helically packaged ribonucleocapsid, which is composed of the genomic RNA intimately associated with protein N, polymerase L and its cofactor protein P (formerly named M1). The ribonucleocapsid complex ensures genome transcription and replication in the cytoplasm.

Finally, protein M (formerly named M2) occupies an intermediate position between the ribonucleocapsid and the envelope, and is responsible for virus budding and the bullet-shaped morphology.

2.2 Demarcation criteria in the *Lyssavirus* genus

Until 1956 and the first isolations of rabies-related viruses in Africa, the rabies virus was believed to be unique and antigenically distinct from other members of the *Rhabdoviridae* family (8). This warranted the creation of the genus *Lyssavirus* (Greek *lyssa*: rabies) for viruses responsible for rabies-like encephalitis. The genus was at first divided into four serotypes (1–4) by antigenic cross-reactivity with sera and monoclonal antibodies, which correspond to the following species: serotype 1, rabies virus (RABV); 2, Lagos bat virus (LBV); 3, Mokola virus (MOKV); and 4, Duvenhage virus (DUVV). Further isolations of new bat lyssaviruses in Europe, then Australia and the progress in genetic characterization of several genes (N, P, and G) supported the delineation of seven genotypes (1–7), confirming and expanding the antigenic data (Table 1): 1, RABV; 2, LBV; 3, MOKV; 4, DUVV; 5, European bat lyssavirus 1 (EBLV-1); 6, European bat lyssavirus 2 (EBLV-2); and 7, Australian bat lyssavirus (ABLV). Within each genotype, sublineages correspond to variants circulating in specific geographical regions and/or animal hosts. The genotypes further segregate in two phylogroups including genotypes 1, 4, 5, 6 and 7 (phylogroup I); and 2 and 3 (phylogroup II). Viruses of each phylogroup differ in their biological properties (pathogenicity, induction of apoptosis, cell receptor recognition, etc.) (9, 10).

It is important to note that bats are reservoirs and vectors for six out of the seven genotypes characterized so far (the precise reservoir/

Table 1

Classification of lyssaviruse

Phylogroup	Genotype	Species	Abbreviation (ICTV)[a]	Geographical origin	Potential vector(s)
Isolates characterized					
I	1	Rabies virus	RABV	Worldwide (except several islands)	Carnivores (worldwide); bats (Americas)
I	4	Duvenhage virus	DUVV	Southern Africa	Insectivorous bats
I	5	European bat lyssavirus type 1	EBLV-1	Europe	Insectivorous bats (*Eptesicus serotinus*)
I	6	European bat lyssavirus type 2	EBLV-2	Europe	Insectivorous bats (*Myotis* sp.)
I	7	Australian bat lyssavirus	ABLV	Australia	Frugivorous/insectivorous bats (*Megachiroptera/Microchiroptera*)
II	2	Lagos bat virus	LBV	Sub-Saharan Africa	Frugivorous bats (*Megachiroptera*)
II	3	Mokola virus	MOKV	Sub-Saharan Africa	Unknown
Isolates to be characterized as new genotypes					
	—	Aravan virus	ARAV	Central Asia	Insectivorous bats (isolated from *Myotis blythi*)
	—	Khujand virus	KHUV	Central Asia	Insectivorous bats (isolated from *Myotis mystacinus*)
	—	Irkut virus	IRKV	East Siberia	Insectivorous bats (isolated from *Murina leucogaster*)
	—	West Caucasian bat virus	WCBV	Caucasian region	Insectivorous bats (isolated from *Miniopterus schreibersi*)

[a] ICTV = International Committee on Taxonomy of Viruses.

vector for genotype 3, MOKV, remains to be determined). For five genotypes, bats are the exclusive vectors, and only genotype 1, RABV, also includes terrestrial vectors (mainly carnivores). Genotype 1 corresponds to the classical rabies virus and is spread in domestic or wild animals worldwide. Genotypes 2–7 have a narrower geographical and host-range distribution (so far, most are confined to the Old World plus Australia).

This classification will evolve, particularly as surveillance for bat lyssaviruses is reinforced (*11*). Four recent isolates of bat lyssavirus in Central Asia, East Siberia and the Caucasian region need to be characterized as new genotypes (Table 1): Aravan virus (ARAV), Khujand virus (KHUV), Irkut virus (IRKV) and West Caucasian bat virus (WCBV).

Lyssaviruses show a broad antigenic cross-reactivity at the nucleocapsid level, mainly because of sequence conservation of the N protein: amino acid identities range from 78% (MOKV and EBLV-2) to 93% (DUVV and EBLV-1). This allows the use of similar reagents for diagnosis by immunofluorescence. The ectodomain of the G protein (carrying the main antigenic sites) is more variable and cross-neutralization exists among lyssaviruses of the same phylogroup (amino acid identities in the ectodomain > 74%), but not between phylogroups (amino acid identities in the ectodomain < 62%). Experimental evidence obtained so far indicates that vaccine strains (all belonging to genotype 1 within phylogroup I) are ineffective for protection against infection by lyssaviruses from phylogroup II.

3. Pathogenesis and diagnosis

3.1 Pathogenesis

Rabies virus entry occurs through wounds or direct contact with mucosal surfaces. The virus cannot cross intact skin. The virus then either replicates in non-nervous tissues or directly enters peripheral nerves and travels by retrograde axoplasmic flow to the central nervous system (CNS). Both motor and sensory fibres may be involved depending on the animal species. The incubation period varies from 2 weeks to 6 years (average 2–3 months) depending on the amount of virus in the inoculum and site of inoculation. The proximity of the site of virus entry to the CNS increases the likelihood of a short incubation period. The estimated speed of virus migration is 15–100 mm per day. The virus then moves from the CNS via anterograde axoplasmic flow within peripheral nerves, leading to infection of some of the adjacent non-nervous tissues: for example, secretory tissues of salivary glands. The virus is widely disseminated throughout the body at the time of clinical onset. The first clinical symptom is usually neuropathic pain at the wound site. This is caused by virus replication in dorsal root ganglia and ganglionitis. Major clinical signs are related to the virus-induced encephalomyeloradiculitis. Two major clinical presentations are observed: furious and paralytic forms that cannot be correlated with any specific anatomical localization of rabies virus in the CNS (12). Nevertheless, peripheral nerve dysfunction is responsible for weakness in paralytic rabies. In furious rabies electrophysiological studies indicate anterior horn cell dysfunction even in the absence of clinical weakness. Without intensive care, death occurs within a few days (1–5 days) of the development of neurological signs. Rabies is inevitably fatal.

3.2 Diagnosis

3.2.1 Clinical diagnosis in humans

Diagnosis of rabies based on clinical grounds alone is difficult and unreliable except when specific clinical signs of hydro- or aerophobia are present. Some patients present with a paralytic or Guillain-Barre-like syndrome or other atypical clinical features (13). Detailed clinical information of atypical rabies patients especially those associated with bat or other wildlife can be accessed through the web site of the United States National Center for Infectious Diseases, Centres for Disease Control and Prevention.[1] Classical signs of brain involvement include spasms in response to tactile, auditory, visual or olfactory stimuli (e.g. aerophobia and hydrophobia) alternating with periods of lucidity, agitation, confusion, and signs of autonomic dysfunction. These spasms occur at some time in almost all rabid patients in whom excitation is prominent. However, spontaneous inspiratory spasms usually occur continuously until death and their presence often facilitates clinical diagnosis. Excitation is less evident in paralytic rabies, and phobic spasms appear in only 50% of these patients. During the early stages of paralytic rabies, notable signs include myoedema at percussion sites, usually in the region of the chest, deltoid muscle and thigh, and piloerection. Atypical or non-classic rabies is being increasingly recognized and may be responsible for underreporting.

Magnetic resonance imaging performed with adequate precautions suitable for potentially infectious patients, can be helpful in diagnoses (14). Abnormal, ill-defined, mildly hypersignal T2 images involving the brainstem, hippocampus, hypothalamus, deep and subcortical

---

[1] http://www.cdc.gov/ncidod

white matter, and deep and cortical grey matter are indicative of rabies, when present, regardless of clinical types. Gadolinium enhancement is clearly shown only in later stages when patients lapse into a coma. Such a pattern differentiates rabies from other viral encephalitides, not in terms of location, but in the T2 image appearance and in the pattern of contrast enhancement when compared according to consciousness status. Computerized tomography of the brain is of no diagnostic value.

Since imported cases of human and animal rabies have been noted in rabies-free countries (or rabies-free areas of infected countries), the Consultation emphasized that rabies must be included in the differential diagnosis of all people who present with signs of encephalitis.

3.2.2 *Laboratory diagnosis*

Definite diagnosis of rabies can only be obtained by laboratory investigations.

Biosafety considerations
Rabies has the highest case-fatality rate of any currently recognized infectious disease. Safety is of paramount importance when working with lyssaviruses.

In general, biosafety level 2 safety practices are adequate for routine laboratory activities such as diagnosis and animal handling. Besides basic facility design, precautions should also include personal protection equipment (e.g. clothing) and pre-exposure vaccination. Certain situations may entail consideration of a biosafety level 3 classification, including production of large quantities of concentrated virus, conducting procedures that may generate aerosols and when working with lyssaviruses for which the effectiveness of current prophylaxis is not known. All national safety guidelines for working with infectious agents should be followed.

Transport of specimens
Specimens for rabies diagnosis should be shipped according to the national and international regulations to avoid exposure hazards. Information on classification (UN 2814) and packing instructions (P620 packaging) can be found in *Transport of infectious substances* (*15*). Diagnostic specimens should either be refrigerated or shipped at room temperature in 50% glycerine-saline solution.

Source of specimens for diagnosis and storage conditions
Rabies diagnosis can be performed on fresh specimens from several different tissue sources or on appropriate specimens stored at proper

temperatures, preferably refrigerated. The choice of specimens depends on the test to be performed and the stage of the disease in humans.

Formalin fixation of brain tissues is not recommended. If specimens are nevertheless received in formalin, the duration of fixation should be less than 7 days. The specimens should be transferred rapidly to absolute ethanol for subsequent molecular diagnosis.

Sampling for intra vitam diagnosis
Secretions and biological fluids (saliva, spinal fluid, tears, etc.) and tissues can be used to diagnose rabies during life (intra vitam). They should be stored at −20 °C or below. Serum should be collected from blood samples prior to freezing and stored at −20 °C or below.

Sampling for postmortem diagnosis
Brain tissue is the preferred specimen for postmortem diagnosis in both humans and animals. In cases where brain tissue is not available, other tissues may be of diagnostic value. In field studies or when an autopsy cannot be performed, techniques of collecting brain-tissue samples via trans-orbital or trans-foramen magnum route can be used (*16, 17*). The use of glycerine preservation (temperature: +4 °C or −20 °C) or dried smears of brain tissue on filter paper (temperature: +30 °C) also enables safe transportation of infected material.

3.2.3 *Techniques for postmortem diagnosis of rabies in animals and humans*

Techniques are described in the WHO *Laboratory techniques in rabies* (*7*) and the OIE *Manual of diagnostic tests and vaccines for terrestrial animals* (*18*).

Antigen detection
The fluorescent antibody (FA) technique is a rapid and sensitive method for diagnosing rabies infection in animals and humans (*19*). It is the gold standard for rabies diagnosis; however, the accuracy of this test depends upon the expertise of the examiner, and the quality of anti-rabies conjugate and the fluorescence microscope. The test is based upon microscopic examination under ultraviolet light of impressions, smears or frozen sections of tissue after they have been treated with anti-rabies serum or globulin conjugated with fluorescein isothiocyanate. The diagnostic conjugate should be of high quality and the appropriate working dilution must be determined in order to detect the different genotypes of lyssavirus.

Impressions (or smears) of tissue samples from brainstem, thalamus, cerebellum, and the hippocampus (Ammon's horns) are recommended for increased sensitivity of the test.

Detection of lyssavirus nucleocapsid antigen by enzyme-linked immunosorbent assay (ELISA) has been described and used for many years in some laboratories (*19*). It is rapid and can be useful for epidemiological surveys. However, at present this test is not commercially available.

Virus isolation

Virus isolation may be necessary to confirm the results of antigen detection tests and for further characterization of the isolate (*19*). Virus isolation can be performed on neuroblastoma cells or upon intracranial inoculation of mice.

Murine neuroblastoma (NA C1300) cells are more susceptible to field isolates of rabies virus than are other cell lines tested. Virus isolation in cell culture (with neuroblastoma cells) is at least as efficient as mouse inoculation for demonstrating small amounts of rabies virus. It also reduces the time required for diagnosis from 10–15 days for the mouse inoculation test to 1–2 days using neuroblastoma cells. When compared with the FA technique, the gold standard, the sensitivity of virus isolation in neuroblastoma cells is higher than 98%. However, false negative results may be obtained with decomposed brains. Where cell culture facilities are not available, mouse inoculation should be used. The technique is sensitive and robust. If a more rapid answer is necessary, suckling mice (less than 3 days old) are preferred to weanling or adult mice since they are more susceptible to rabies virus. The observation period may be shortened by FA examination of brains of inoculated mice killed 3–4 days (or more) after inoculation.

Detection by molecular techniques

The use of the polymerase chain reaction (PCR) and other amplification techniques is not currently recommended for routine post-mortem diagnosis of rabies. However, these molecular techniques can be applied for epidemiological surveys in laboratories with strict quality control procedures in place and that have experience and expertise with these techniques.

3.2.4 *Techniques for intra vitam diagnosis of rabies in humans*

The sensitivity of techniques for rabies diagnosis varies greatly according to the stage of the disease, antibody status, intermittent nature of viral shedding and the training of the technical staff. While a positive result is indicative of rabies, a negative result does not necessarily rule out the infection. Brain biopsy taken solely for the diagnosis of rabies is not recommended (20).

Antigen detection
Viral antigen may be detected by using the FA test on skin biopsies from patients with clinical rabies. Test results are independent of the antibody status of the patient. Substantial numbers of rabies patients have FA-positive skin specimens during the early phase of the disease. Skin biopsies are usually taken from the nuchal area of the neck, with hair follicles containing peripheral nerves. Examination of at least 20 sections is required to detect rabies nucleocapsid inclusions around the base of hair follicles. The quality of skin biopsy samples is of paramount importance. Though sensitive, this technique may not be practical in all settings, because of the need for a cryostat to prepare frozen tissue sections.

FA testing on corneal impressions is rarely reliable in most clinical settings and is therefore not recommended.

Virus isolation
Rabies virus isolation can be performed using neuroblastoma cells or the intracranial inoculation of mice. Virus isolation is preferably performed on saliva samples or other biological fluids such as tears and cerebrospinal fluid. The success rate depends upon the antibody status (more positive results are obtained in antibody-negative patients) and on the intermittence of viral shedding.

Liquid specimens conserved as such or in swabs should be maintained frozen after collection. The contents of the swab should be expelled into the collection medium. Under no circumstances should preservatives be added to the collection medium.

It should be noted that infectious virus may be absent from these specimens even during the late stage of the disease.

Antibody titration
Neutralizing antibodies in the serum or cerebrospinal fluid of non-vaccinated patients can be measured using a virus neutralization test such as the rapid fluorescent focus inhibition test (RFFIT) or the fluorescent antibody virus neutralization (FAVN) test. Virus-neutralizing antibodies in serum tend to appear on average 8 days after clinical symptoms appear. Rabies antibodies are infrequently found in cerebrospinal fluid.

An ELISA using purified rabies glycoprotein has been used to determine anti-glycoprotein antibody levels in the serum of humans and of some animal species. This assay can be useful when the RFFIT is not available.

Molecular techniques
Molecular detection by polymerase chain reaction and nucleic acid sequence-based amplification techniques has the highest level of sensitivity but requires standardization and very stringent quality control (*21*). Rabies virus RNA can be detected in several biological fluids and samples (e.g. saliva, cerebrospinal fluid, tears, skin biopsy sample and urine). Serial samples of fluids (e.g. saliva and urine) should be tested, owing to intermittent shedding of virus. Such techniques can produce false positive or false negative results, and should only be used in combination with other conventional techniques.

3.2.5 Virus identification using molecular techniques: epidemiological considerations

To date, thousands of lyssavirus isolates from humans and domestic and wild animals have been evaluated and compared using molecular techniques. These studies have permitted the classification of lyssaviruses into genotypes and demonstrated that virus isolates from a given geographical area have unique genetic sequence patterns both in the nucleocapsid and glycoprotein components. In most cases, these differences can also be used to identify the principal reservoir (bat, dog, fox, etc.).

4. Management of rabies patients before and after death

4.1 Treatment of rabies patients

Rabies is a fatal disease. The following measures have been assessed in clinical rabies, but without any evidence of effectiveness: administration of vidarabine, multisite intradermal vaccination with cell-culture vaccine, administration of α-interferon and rabies immunoglobulin by intravenous as well as intrathecal routes, and administration of anti-thymocyte globulin, high doses of steroids, inosine pranobex, ribavirin and high doses of the antibody-binding fragments of rabies immunoglobulin G (*22*).

The clinical course of the disease, with either excitation or paralysis is the predominant symptom, is of short duration and entails much suffering. Patients remain conscious, often aware of the nature of their illness, and are usually extremely agitated, particularly when excitation is predominant. This is compounded by the fact that they become isolated because of the perceived risk of transmission of the virus through contact. Patients with confirmed rabies should receive adequate sedation and comfort care in an appropriate medical facility, preferably in a private room with suitable emotional and physical support. Repeated intravenous morphine has been demonstrated to be effective in relieving severe agitation, anxiety, and phobic spasms that afflict furious rabies patients. Once rabies diagnosis has been confirmed, invasive procedures should be avoided. The patient should be cared for in a private, quiet and draft-free area. Considering the hopelessness of rabies in man, treatment should centre on comfort care; using heavy sedation (barbiturates, morphine) and avoidance of intubation and life-support measures once the diagnosis is certain. As new treatment modalities become evident, specialized centres may wish to institute experimental therapies with informed consent from patient and family. This should be at no cost to the victim's estate. Parties authorized to give permission for such treatment should also be informed that survival is likely to result in severe neurological deficits.

4.2 Transmission via organ transplants

Considering a recent report (May 2004) from the USA of a cluster of human rabies cases associated with transplantation of solid organs from a misdiagnosed rabies patient, the Consultation expressed concern about the risk of transmission of rabies virus through organ transplants (see section 12.1.6).

4.3 Recommendations for safe clinical management of rabies patients

The care of humans diagnosed with rabies often creates great anxiety in a hospital setting, involving not only medical and nursing staff but the media and the public. In fact, human rabies should not pose any greater risk to health-care staff than do most bacterial or other viral infections. However, staff should wear gowns, goggles, masks and gloves. This is particularly important when intubation and suctioning are performed. The virus is not carried in blood and is only intermittently shed in saliva, CNS fluid, urine and within some tissues. Pre-exposure immunization against rabies of nursing staff and health-care personnel in hospitals may be considered for those who, after careful investigation, are considered most at risk. However increasing staff awareness of the need to strictly adhere to proper barrier nursing methods for patient care, as is recommended for all infectious diseases, should be emphasized as equally if not more important in caring for rabies patients.

Specialized centres caring for rabies patients should provide pre-exposure vaccination for health-care staff involved in rabies case management. Some centres have used a shortened pre-exposure immunization regimen consisting of tissue-culture rabies vaccine administered on days 0, 3, 7 and 14.

4.4 Postmortem management of bodies of patients that have died of rabies

Careless handling of brain or spinal cord, such as using electric saws and drills during brain biopsy or necropsy, may be risky. Such procedures should be conducted using goggles and respiratory protection. Tissues and body fluids should be disposed of in the same manner as practiced for other infectious diseases such as tuberculosis and hepatitis.

Humans who have died of rabies generally present a small risk of transmission to others. There is evidence that blood does not contain virus but that the virus is present in many tissues such as the CNS, salivary glands and muscle. It can also be present in saliva and urine. Embalming should be discouraged. Performing necropsies carelessly can lead to mucous membrane and inhalation exposures. Wearing protective clothing, goggles, a face mask and thick gloves should provide sufficient protection. Instruments must be autoclaved or boiled after use. Early disposal of the body by cremation or burial is recommended.

5. Rabies vaccines and immunoglobulins

Several strains of fixed rabies virus were recommended previously by WHO for human and animal vaccine production, and experience over the past decade has established their safety, antigenicity and efficacy. They are:

— Pasteur (Paris) virus strains (PV, for Pasteur virus) of rabbit fixed rabies virus; also adapted to Vero cells;
— PV-12 strain of Pasteur rabbit fixed rabies virus; also adapted to BHK-21 cells;
— Pitman-Moore (PM) strain of fixed rabies virus, adapted to human diploid, primary dog kidney and Vero cells;
— CVS (challenge virus strain)-11 Kissling strain, adapted to BHK-21 cells;
— LEP (low egg passage) (40–50 passages) Flury chick embryo-adapted rabies virus, also adapted to primary chick embryo cells and to BHK-21 cells;

— HEP (high egg passage) (227–230 passages) Flury chick embryo-adapted rabies virus; also adapted to primary chick embryo cells;
— Kelev (100 passages) chick embryo-adapted rabies virus;
— ERA (Evelyn Rokitniki Abelseth) strain of Street-Alabama-Dufferin (SAD) virus, adapted to porcine kidney cells; also adapted to BHK-21 cells (in Canada);
— different SAD variants are ERA virus adapted to BHK-21 cells (in Europe).

Vaccine strains may be obtained through WHO upon request provided conditions regarding, in particular, their production and accessibility to patients are fulfilled and shipment costs are covered by the recipient laboratory.

5.1 Rabies vaccines for humans

5.1.1 *Human vaccine types*

Considerable progress has been made in the production and use of rabies vaccines in the past two decades. Various safe regimens have been developed to reduce the cost of active immunization. Over the past 20 years, many developing countries have discontinued the production and use of brain-tissue vaccines for human use and have managed to meet their needs by importing vaccine. Other countries have developed or acquired modern technology for the production of cell-culture rabies vaccines. All vaccines produced in nerve tissues have been found to be reactogenic and some are of low immunogenicity. The Consultation strongly recommends that nerve-tissue vaccines should be discontinued. Only cell-culture and purified embryonated egg vaccines should be used in humans. Rabies vaccines for human use should meet WHO requirements for the production and control of such vaccines, as well as the recommendations and guidelines that apply to the production of rabies vaccines (*23–29*). WHO requirements for production and control of rabies vaccines for human use are currently under revision. More details regarding the revision can be found in the meeting reports from 2003 and 2004 (*30, 31*); the latest information is available on the WHO web site.[1]

Virus strains used for vaccine production must be carefully selected and periodic evaluation of the antigenic identity of the virus strains as well as the identity and purity of the cell lines used for production should be conducted. Virus strains used in vaccine production must be proven to be protective against the viruses circulating in the areas where they will be used.

---

[1] http://www.who.int/biologicals/publications/meetings/areas/vaccines/rabies

A description of the production techniques for several vaccines has been previously published in *Laboratory techniques in rabies* (*7*).

There are multiple reasons why nerve-tissue vaccines have not been replaced as has been recommended by the WHO Expert Committee on Rabies in its seventh (*32*), and eighth (*1*) reports. These reasons may include the perceived high cost of switching production technology and of licensing of cell-culture rabies vaccines. During any transition periods, vaccine availability must be ensured.

When technology transfer occurs, vaccines must meet WHO requirements for production and control.

5.1.2 *Potency requirements for human vaccines*

As rabies is a fatal disease, it is absolutely essential that every batch of vaccine released is of adequate potency. The test that is currently used to assess vaccine potency is the National Institutes of Health (NIH) test as described in *Laboratory techniques in rabies* (*7*). The minimum potency required for all cell-culture and purified embryonated egg rabies vaccines is 2.5 international units (IU) per single intramuscular dose.

General principles for clinical evaluation of vaccines, which also apply to rabies vaccines, are available in the WHO guidelines for clinical evaluation of vaccines (*33*). In addition, a number of recommendations for non-clinical evaluation of vaccines should also be consulted since non-clinical testing is a prerequisite to the initiation of clinical trials (*34*).

5.1.3 *Failure of vaccines and full post-exposure prophylaxis*

All failures of vaccines and combined vaccine and immunoglobulin post-exposure prophylaxis should be investigated thoroughly and independently to identify potential errors in treatment protocol, low vaccine potency, immunocompromised patients, and/or newly emerging or previously unknown rabies virus variants. A national vaccine adverse-event reporting system should be established. Post-marketing surveillance for vaccine and immunoglobulin efficacy and safety in the field should be in place (see Annex 5).

5.1.4 *Routes of administration*

WHO recommends one intramuscular and one intradermal regimen for pre-exposure immunization (see section 6.1), two intramuscular regimens and two intradermal regimens for post-exposure prophylaxis (see section 6.2 and Annex 1).

Considering the recommendations on intradermal application of rabies vaccines in the eighth report of the WHO Expert Committee on Rabies published in 1992 (*1*), a number of WHO consultations have contributed over time to the further assessment and wider use of reduced dosage intradermal vaccination regimens for rabies pre- and post-exposure prophylaxis. These regimens consist of the intradermal administration of a fraction of the intramuscular dose of certain rabies vaccines at multiple sites (*35–37*). The regimens are described in details in Annex 1. Only two commercial products are today considered safe and efficacious by WHO for use by the intradermal route (see Annex 1).

The use of this route leads to considerable savings in terms of the total amount of vaccine needed for a full pre- or post-exposure vaccination series, thereby reducing the cost of active immunization.

These intradermal regimens are of particular interest in areas where rabies vaccines are in short supply or available but inaccessible, in view of their price, to people at risk of contracting rabies. The intradermal route for rabies vaccine administration should advantageously replace post-exposure prophylaxis using brain-tissue vaccines in all countries where these vaccines are still produced and usually administered to the poorest segment of the population.

The decision to implement economical intradermal post-exposure prophylaxis rests with government agencies that define rabies prevention and treatment policies in their own countries. When the intradermal route is used, precautions include staff training, conditions and duration of vaccine storage after reconstitution, use of appropriate 1 ml syringe and short hypodermic needles. Vaccines to be applied by intradermal route of administration should meet WHO requirements for production and control related to vaccines for intramuscular use, including an NIH test potency of at least 2.5 IU per single (intramuscular) dose. In addition, immunogenicity and safety of the vaccine in question should be demonstrated in appropriate human trials using WHO post-exposure prophylaxis regimens. In countries where relevant national authorities have approved the intradermal route for rabies pre- and/or post-exposure prophylaxis, and for vaccines that can be used by that route, the vaccine package leaflet should include a statement indicating that the potency as well as immunogenicity and safety allow safe use of the vaccine for intradermal pre- and post-exposure prophylaxis, in addition to other relevant information as described in the WHO requirements for vaccine production and control.

5.2 Vaccines for animals

5.2.1 *Animal vaccine types*

Injectable animal vaccines

Modified live-virus vaccines

Modified live-virus vaccines are not recommended for use for parenteral immunization; rabies infection can occur as a result of the vaccine strain.

Cell-culture vaccines

Inactivated vaccines can be produced in cell culture, using either primary cells or continuous cell lines. The seed virus/cell systems vary considerably between different manufacturers. Improvements in vaccine production techniques during the last decade have led to an increased use of inactivated adjuvanted vaccines for animal immunization.

The duration of immunity and safety are especially important when a vaccine is being selected for use in a mass vaccination campaign. Use of vaccines that will provide stable and long-lasting immunity is recommended, because this constitutes the most effective method of controlling and eliminating the disease in animals. Regardless of the vaccine used, it must be administered properly to provide the desired protection.

Nerve-tissue vaccines

Inactivated nerve-tissue vaccines can be produced from the brains of lambs or suckling mice. Such vaccines have been shown to be effective in mass canine immunization programmes in North Africa (lamb brain vaccines) as well as in Latin America and the Caribbean (suckling-mouse brain vaccines). In the future, because of the availability of safe and inexpensive locally produced cell-culture vaccines, replacement of all nerve-tissue rabies vaccines with cell-culture vaccines can be expected.

Combined vaccines

Use of combined vaccines will certainly lead to a wider range of immunoprophylactic strategies against different microbial pathogens, and has already simplified the vaccination schedule. No indication of competitive inhibition of the immune response has been reported for combined vaccines, but each new product should be investigated for its overall immunogenic potency. Attention should be paid to all vaccine components, including rabies antigen.

Combined rabies vaccines are already used for the immunization of dogs and cats. Several different antigens have been incorporated into canine rabies vaccines, such as canine distemper virus, canine adenovirus type 1, *Leptospira* and canine parvovirus. Combined vaccines currently available for cats include various antigens such as feline panleukopenia virus, feline calicivirus and feline parvoviruses. A combined rabies and foot-and-mouth disease vaccine is available for use in cattle, sheep and goats.

Oral animal vaccines

Modified live-virus vaccines

Several types of modified live-virus vaccines with various levels of attenuation have been developed for oral immunization of wildlife. SAD B19 and SAD P5/88 vaccines are produced by several cell-culture passages of the SAD Berne strain, which is a cell culture-adapted derivative of the ERA strain. The SAG (Street Alabama Gif) 2 vaccine was selected from the SAD Berne strain after two successive mutations of the arginine 333 codon were performed using selected monoclonal antibodies.

SAD-related vaccines have been widely used in the field in both Europe and Canada. Between 1978 and the early 1990s, a large number of SAD-related vaccine baits were distributed in several European countries for the control of fox rabies, as well as in another European country to combat racoon dog rabies. While some of these countries opted later for alternative vaccine types, the use of SAD-related vaccines was extended to other parts of eastern Europe. The rabies situation has improved drastically in certain of these countries, such as the Czech Republic, which has not reported any cases of rabies during the past two years, and in Austria, which has reported no cases during 2004, as well as in the Ontario province of Canada.

No adverse effects following the oral administration of 10 times the field dose of SAG2 were reported in target species (red fox, dog, raccoon dog and arctic fox) or in non-target species including: baboons; six different rodents species including rats; two species of corvids; wild boars, badgers, goats, ferrets, hedgehogs and diurnal and nocturnal prey birds. During a recent trial conducted in India on caged street dogs, no adverse effects were observed in any dog, even those immunosuppressed, that received freeze-dried SAG2 in administered baits. In efficacy studies, red foxes (adult and cubs), raccoon dogs and dogs were protected from virulent challenge after immunization with one single SAG2 bait. No salivary excretion of infective

SAG2 virus strain was detected in dogs after vaccination. In bait, SAG2 is either contained in a capsule as a viral suspension or incorporated in the bait matrix as a freeze-dried suspension, for use in countries with canine rabies.

Live recombinant vaccines

A recombinant vaccinia virus expressing the glycoprotein gene of rabies virus (VRG) was developed by inserting the cDNA of the glycoprotein of ERA strain into the thymidine kinase gene of vaccinia virus (Copenhagen strain). When administered orally (by direct instillation into the oral cavity or in a bait), a dose of 10^8 TCID$_{50}$ (median tissue-culture infective dose) of VRG elicits titres of virus neutralizing antibodies and confers a protective immune response against rabies virus challenge in a number of carnivorous or omnivorous mammalian species (red fox, arctic fox, coyote, raccoon, raccoon dog, domestic dog and golden jackal). In the field, the VRG vaccine strain is stable above 56 °C and the bait-casing melting point is above 60 °C.

The recombinant virus expressing VRG does not exhibit residual pathogenicity caused by rabies, however it shares basic properties with its parental virus, the human smallpox vaccine strain vaccinia Copenhagen. As shown in the severely compromised immune deficient mouse model, insertion of the rabies glycoprotein gene into the thymidine kinase locus attenuates the recombinant compared with the parental strain. Safety studies conducted in over 50 mammalian and 10 avian species, many of which are major rabies vectors, have not revealed any residual pathogenicity. One clinical adverse reaction has been documented in humans. It involved spontaneously cleared skin lesions in a person with assumed increased susceptibility to the vaccinia virus, as a result of exposure to the vaccine, through a bite while attempting to remove a partially chewed vaccine bait from a dog's mouth.

VRG has been used to successfully control or reduce wildlife or canine rabies in a variety of animal species such as red foxes (Belgium, France, Israel, Luxemburg), raccoon dogs (Republic of Korea), coyotes, raccoons and grey foxes (Canada and USA) and experimentally in domestic dogs (Sri Lanka) (38).

5.2.2 *Potency requirements for animal vaccines*

Inactivated animal rabies vaccines

The Consultation suggested that inactivated animal vaccines with a potency of less than 1.0 IU per dose, as measured by the NIH test or other recognized pharmacopoeia tests, should not be licensed or released unless an adequately designed experiment has demonstrated a duration of protection of at least 1 year in the species for which the vaccine is to be used.

The potency of inactivated parenteral vaccines should be ascertained at intervals after they have been distributed. Inactivated vaccine, even in liquid form, is relatively stable when stored under proper conditions. To verify that storage conditions are adequate, it is recommended that samples from the field that are approaching their expiry date be tested using the methods applied to newly manufactured products (*33*).

Animal rabies vaccines for oral immunization

Minimum potency requirements for oral vaccines for immunization of wild animals have not been established, although the median effective doses (ED_{50}) of various modified live-virus and recombinant vaccines are known. Minimum potency requirements for oral vaccines intended to immunize wild animals are of importance since numerous studies have demonstrated that the level of protection is correlated with the virus titre. The batch releasing titre should correspond to at least 10 times the 100% protective dose.

To test the efficacy of candidate vaccines for oral immunization, sufficient numbers of target animals should be maintained under captive conditions, given the vaccine and challenged with rabies virus. The potency of the vaccines should be standardized to quantifiable levels (e.g. plaque-forming units/ml, $TCID_{50}$/ml). Once efficacy has been demonstrated under laboratory conditions in the target species, the vaccine should be administered in a bait identical to that to be used in field trials. Serial dilutions of test vaccine will determine the ED_{50}. Animals should then be held for a minimum of 6–12 months prior to a challenge with a field strain of rabies virus administered by the intramuscular route; the interval between vaccine administration and challenge is dependent upon the turnover rate of the target species. Potency estimates should not be based entirely on the ability of the vaccine to induce virus-neutralizing antibodies in the target species; environmental stability tests are also necessary to demonstrate that vaccine potency is retained under field conditions (see section 7).

Thermostability of the bait casing is also essential to ensure that the capsule of the vaccine is still covered if exposed to high field temperatures, thus ensuring virus titre stability. Most rabies vaccine baits disappear within 7 days after distribution in the fields, considerably reducing potential biohazardous waste.

5.2.3 *Safety of animal vaccines*

Vaccines for parenteral use

Several types of safety tests for inactivated rabies vaccines have been proposed. They are described in *Laboratory techniques in rabies* (7) and the *Manual of diagnostic tests and vaccines for terrestrial animals* (*18*).

In view of the hazard of encephalitogenic reactions, discontinuation of nerve-tissue vaccines should be considered. The absence of live virus in inactivated vaccines must be confirmed by the most sensitive assays available.

The finished vaccine must not contain detectable levels of β-propiolactone or any other inactivating agent, except in the case of Semple vaccine, where phenol may be allowed in the final product.

The Consultation recommended that purity testing should encompass not only the seed virus material but also the cell cultures and other biological ingredients used in vaccine manufacture. The Consultation recommended that new rabies vaccines for animals be tested for safety by direct inoculation in the species for which they are to be used. The numbers of animals available for this type of testing will ordinarily be insufficient to demonstrate unusual virus–host reactions, and any reported vaccine-associated problems arising during field use should be reported to the appropriate national and international authorities and rigorously investigated.

Vaccines for oral immunization

The vaccine strain should be characterized according to procedures recommended for rabies vaccines for veterinary use and according to international guidelines (*39, 40*).

The safety of vaccines is assessed in target and non-target species, namely wild rodents and other wild and domestic species, and also in non-human primates.

The vaccines have different residual pathogenicity related to the level of attenuation of the viral strain. The SAD strains appear to be pathogenic for adult mice and other rodent species irrespective of the route of inoculation (intracerebral, intramuscular or oral). The SAD Berne strain is pathogenic for the baboon by the oral route.

The SAG2 and VRG vaccines are not pathogenic for adult mice and several other wild rodents tested by the oral, intramuscular or intra-cerebral routes. Additionally, several studies have demonstrated that these vaccines are not pathogenic for a large number of mammalian species, including the majority of reservoir hosts.

The possibility of excretion of candidate vaccine virus in the saliva of the target species should be examined. No virus should be detectable after a maximum of 3–4 days following immunization. Any virus that is recovered should be characterized using molecular techniques or monoclonal antibodies. Reduced levels of vaccine virus excretion are important to reduce opportunities for non-target species (including humans) contamination. Only vaccines with the lowest known re-sidual pathogenicity (SAG2 and VRG) should be used in dogs.

The vaccine chosen for use should not produce any disease when administered orally at 10 times the dose recommended for field use in at least 10 young (3–6 months old) animals of the target species, or in dogs less than 10 weeks of age (*40*).

In addition, where feasible, at least 10 and if possible 50 of each of the most common local rodent species should be given the field dose of vaccine (i.e. the dose which is contained in a bait) orally and intramus-cularly (this may require use of different virus concentrations and volumes for different species, depending on their weight and size). If the animals that are vaccinated become sick or die from rabies, the use of the vaccine should be re-evaluated.

Relevant local wild or domestic animal species that may consume baits should also be administered the field dose of vaccine orally in a volume adapted to body weight (*41*, *42*).

Any rabies virus isolated from animals in vaccination areas should be characterized using monoclonal antibodies or molecular techniques to ensure that no vaccine-induced rabies has occurred.

5.3 Rabies immunoglobulins

There are three classes of rabies biologicals currently available for passive immunization: human rabies immunoglobulin (HRIG), equine rabies immunoglobulins (ERIG), and highly purified F(ab′)2 products produced from ERIG. They are described, with the modalities of their application, in Annex 1. Possible adverse reactions following their use in humans are also described in section 6.2.3.

Their use in animals is discouraged.

6. Prevention of rabies in humans

Vaccines used for the prevention of rabies in humans, including both pre- and post-exposure prophylaxis, should always meet WHO recommendations for production and control (23-26). Treatment for the prevention of rabies in humans exposed to rabies should begin as soon as possible after the exposure occurs. Treatment consists of thorough wound cleansing for a minimum of 15 minutes using water, soap and a virucidal antiseptic (e.g. povidone iodine or ethanol) followed by the administration of rabies passive immunization and cell-culture or purified embryonated egg rabies vaccine of proven efficacy. The initial treatment of severely exposed (category III) subjects must include injection of rabies immunoglobulin according to WHO recommendations (see Annex 1). The Consultation strongly advocates the use of cell-culture or purified embryonated egg rabies vaccines that comply with WHO criteria for potency, immunogenicity, innocuity, and safety that have been satisfactorily assessed in well-designed clinical trials.

6.1 Pre-exposure vaccination

National authorities should provide guidance as to who should receive pre-exposure vaccination. Generally pre-exposure vaccination should be offered to people at high risk of exposure such as those working in rabies diagnostic or research laboratories, veterinarians, animal handlers (including bat handlers), animal rehabilitators and wildlife officers, as well as other people (especially children) living in or travelling to high-risk areas. Children under 15 years of age are the most frequently exposed age group, representing approximately 50% of human exposures in canine rabies-infected areas. Vaccines produced in cell culture or from embryonated eggs should be used for pre-exposure vaccination of humans. Pre-exposure vaccination is administered as one full dose of vaccine intramuscularly or 0.1 ml intradermally on days 0, 7 and either day 21 or 28. A few days' variation is acceptable. Vaccine is administered into the upper arm (deltoid region) of adults and into the anterolateral thigh region of young children. Vaccine should never be administered into the gluteal region as absorption is unpredictable. Rabies vaccines having a potency of at least 2.5 IU per single intramuscular dose (NIH test) will induce long-lasting memory cells causing an accelerated immune response when a booster dose of vaccine is administered. People currently receiving malaria prophylaxis or who are unable to complete the entire three-dose pre-exposure series prior to initiation of malarial prophylaxis should receive pre-exposure vaccination by the intramuscular route. If the immune status of a patient is questionable at the time of vaccination, his or her immune response to the vaccine should be assessed after the three-dose pre-exposure series has been administered.

Periodic booster injections are recommended for people who are at continual risk of rabies exposure. The following guidelines are recommended for determining when boosters should be administered.

— All people who work with live rabies virus in a diagnostic or research laboratory or in vaccine production should have periodic antibody determinations to avoid unnecessary boosters.
— People at continuous risk, e.g. rabies researchers, diagnostic laboratory workers (where virus is present continuously, often in high concentrations, and where specific exposures are likely to go unrecognized) should have serological testing every 6 months. Judging the relative risk of exposure and the monitoring of vaccination status is the responsibility of the laboratory supervisor. A booster is recommended if the titre falls below 0.5 IU/ml.
— Responsible authorities should ensure that all people at risk are vaccinated and that serological status is monitored.

A rabies pre-exposure certificate should be completed and given to the vaccinee indicating the type of vaccine and vaccine regimen used, lot number of vaccine, and any adverse reactions that occurred during vaccination (see Annex 2).

6.2 Post-exposure prophylaxis

6.2.1 General considerations

All people exposed to rabies should promptly and thoroughly cleanse their wound(s) and apply appropriate antiseptics. Professional assistance is advised. This should be followed, if careful medical assessment requires it, by a complete vaccine series using a potent and effective vaccine that meets WHO criteria and passive immunization for category III exposures. A complete guide to post-exposure prophylaxis can be found in Annex 1. Strict adherence to the WHO-recommended guidelines for optimal post-exposure rabies prophylaxis virtually guarantees protection from the disease. Rabies vaccines for human use that meet WHO requirements for production and control are safe and effective and are free from the neuroparalytic adverse reactions associated with nerve tissue-derived products. Pregnancy, infancy, old age and concurrent illness are not contraindications for rabies post-exposure prophylaxis in the event of an exposure. Prolonged incubation periods have been associated with human rabies; therefore people who present for treatment even months after a possible rabies exposure should be evaluated and treated as if the event had occurred recently.

Factors that should be considered in deciding whether or not to initiate post-exposure prophylaxis include:

- nature of the contact or injury;
- presence of rabies in the area where the contact occurred or where the animal responsible originated;
- availability of the animal for laboratory examination or observation;
- species of the animal;
- clinical status of the animal responsible;
- vaccination history of the animal, and type and timing of vaccine used.

The decision to administer post-exposure prophylaxis after an exposure to an apparently healthy animal should be based on a careful risk assessment by a qualified medical professional. The risk assessment should consider the criteria outlined above. A history of rabies vaccination in an animal is not always a guarantee that the biting animal is not rabid. Animal vaccine failures may occur because of improper administration or poor quality of the vaccine, poor health status of the animal, and the fact that one vaccine dose does not always provide long-lasting protection against infection in dogs. Whether a dog bite was provoked rather than unprovoked should not be considered a guarantee that the animal is not rabid as it can be difficult to understand what an attacking dog considers provocation for an attack. If the animal involved in the exposure is a potential rabies vector in a rabies-endemic region, initiation of post-exposure prophylaxis should never await the results of laboratory examination, nor should the responsible animal be observed for signs of rabies prior to starting post-exposure prophylaxis. Wound treatment and administration of rabies biologicals, including a passive immunization product, when required, and vaccine, should be started as soon as possible after exposure. Immediate humane killing of the animal and examination of the brain at a reliable laboratory should be performed whenever possible. If the species involved is unlikely to be infected with rabies, treatment may be deferred pending the outcome of laboratory testing, providing that results can be obtained within 48 hours.

If the attacking animal is a pet dog or cat that is available, it should be kept under observation for 10 days, preferably under the supervision of a veterinarian. Prophylaxis can be discontinued if the dog or cat remains healthy for at least 10 days after the exposure occurred (*43*, *44*). The natural history of rabies in mammals other than dogs or cats is not fully understood and therefore the 10-day observation period may not be applicable. Humans exposed to other species of mammals suspected to be rabid, including bats and other wild animals involved in the transmission of rabies should therefore receive post-exposure prophylaxis unless the animal can be captured, humanely killed and immediately examined at a reliable laboratory.

6.2.2 *Certificate of post-exposure prophylaxis*

A certificate of post-exposure prophylaxis should be filled in and given to each vaccinee (see Annex 2).

6.2.3 *Complications of post-exposure prophylaxis*

Rabies immunoglobulins
Early local injection-site reactions consisting of erythema and itching are not uncommon with both human and purified equine immunoglobulins. Published data indicate that immunoglobulins can be safely injected into already infected animal bite wounds following proper wound cleansing and the administration of appropriate antibiotics.

Equine rabies immunoglobulin

Most ERIGs that are manufactured presently are highly purified and the occurrence of adverse events has been significantly reduced. Unlike the original unpurified rabies antisera which resulted in adverse reactions in as many as 40% of recipients, the adverse-reaction rate of patients receiving highly purified ERIGs has been reduced to <1–2%. Serious adverse reactions, including anaphylaxis, may occur in spite of a negative skin test. ERIG should only be used by medical staff trained and equipped to manage such an adverse reaction. Unpurified rabies antisera are not recommended.

F(ab′)2 products

F(ab′)2 fragments are obtained by cleavage of the immunoglobulin by a proteolytic enzyme, pepsin, followed by separation of the F(ab′)2 fragments from the Fc fragment. Many of the ERIGs now available are produced in this way.

F(ab′)2 fragments are cleared more rapidly in vivo than intact immunoglobulins. Undesirable side-effects are rare and are similar to those listed above for ERIGs.

Human rabies immunoglobulin

HRIG produced under good manufacturing practices is virtually devoid of serious adverse reactions. It is purified from carefully selected donors, and processing eliminates viral contaminants including those of the human immunodeficiency and hepatitis viruses.

Purified cell-culture and embryonated egg rabies vaccines

These vaccines have not been causally associated with serious adverse effects. Mild serum sickness-like and urticarial reactions have been occasionally been observed following booster doses of human diploid cell vaccine.

7. National programmes for the control of rabies in dogs

Canine rabies can be eliminated, as has been demonstrated in North America, western Europe, Japan and many areas in South America. However, canine rabies is still widespread, occurring in over 80 countries and territories, which are predominantly in the developing world. In more than 99% of all human rabies cases, the virus is transmitted from dogs; half of the global human population lives in canine rabies-endemic areas and is considered at risk of contracting rabies.

Effective animal vaccines that provide a considerable duration of immunity have been developed and mass parenteral vaccination programmes remain the mainstay of canine rabies control. Dog destruction alone is not effective in rabies control.

The principal challenge is effective delivery of vaccines to ensure adequate vaccination coverage in the reservoir dog population. Studies coordinated by WHO on dog populations have shown that, in many communities in Africa, Latin America and Asia (45), a substantial proportion (at least 60–75%) of the total dog population is accessible for parenteral immunization. In communities where dogs are less accessible (for example, in areas with large populations of ownerless dogs), oral rabies vaccination may provide a potential supplementary strategy. Vaccination coverage of 70% has been sufficient to control canine rabies in several settings, but the exact level of coverage required is likely to vary according to the demographic, behavioural and spatial characteristics of the dog population.

During the last two decades, a significant reduction in human rabies has been achieved in Mexico, South America and the Caribbean by the programme for the elimination of canine rabies initiated and coordinated by the Pan American Health Organization/WHO Regional Office for the Americas. In contrast, over the past two decades rabies has been increasing in parts of sub-Saharan Africa and Asia, attributed to rapidly growing dog populations and increasing urbanization, density and mobility of human populations.

To ensure effective coverage, vaccination programmes should consider the local ecology of the dog population, involve coordination of related sectors and incorporate culturally appropriate education efforts. Key to the success of campaigns in Latin America has been the central role played by the public health sector as a lead agency and community/involvement/empowerment in rabies control activities.

Canine rabies control programmes should incorporate three basic elements, with priorities varying according to the prevailing social, cultural and economic factors. The basic elements are: (a) epidemiological surveillance (section 7.1); (b) mass vaccination (section 7.2); and (c) dog population control (section 7.3 and 7.4). They require community participation, managerial skills and legislation.

7.1 Epidemiological surveillance

Rabies should be a notifiable disease within national health and veterinary systems. Rabies surveillance is still inadequate in many countries and this deficit should be addressed by national authorities, with the support of international agencies. Rabies can only be reliably diagnosed by laboratory tests and it is strongly recommended that, in countries where diagnostic facilities are inadequate or lacking, laboratory capacity be developed to permit effective rabies surveillance.

Epidemiological data should be collected, processed, analysed and disseminated rapidly between sectors and different administrative levels. Surveillance of rabies is the basis for any programme of rabies control. Veterinary surveillance of rabies and laboratory submission of reports of suspected animal cases is also essential for management of potential human exposures and for veterinarians to adopt appropriate measures towards animals in contact with a suspected animal case.

The emphasis of surveillance should be on the laboratory confirmation and effective reporting of human and animal rabies cases. Surveillance of areas in which laboratory-confirmed cases in animals are reported should be encouraged. Attempts should be made to isolate viruses for characterization of prevalent strains. This work should be carried out in designated and well-equipped provincial, national or regional laboratories.

Reporting of laboratory-confirmed human rabies cases alone may lead to a severe underestimation of the true number of human cases, resulting in a low priority being given to rabies control. Therefore data on the number of humans suspected as being rabid based on clinical evaluation should also be reported. The number of people seeking and receiving post-exposure prophylaxis should be reported in order to provide additional epidemiological information on disease burden and to evaluate the effectiveness and cost–benefit of rabies control programmes. These data can be compiled from information in the case-record form for human exposure to rabies (see Annex 5).

Countries are urged to adopt or establish systems of rabies reporting (see section 11), especially for the investigation of rabies outbreaks and identification of the rabies virus strains involved, in view of increased international travel and transfer of animals.

7.2 Canine mass parenteral vaccination campaigns

Mass canine vaccination campaigns have been the most effective measure for controlling canine rabies. Since the 1980s, national mass canine vaccination campaigns have been conducted generally on an annual basis in Latin America, with high coverage (around 80%) achieved in a short period of time (no more than 1 week). Over the region, approximately 45 million dogs a year have been vaccinated, resulting in significant declines in canine and human rabies. The organization of the campaigns is based on intersectoral collaboration, community participation and strong media support. Three committees (national, subregional and local) have been established to deal with technical and logistical aspects of the campaigns. The success and sustainability of these campaigns in Latin America have been due to political commitment, acquisition and supply of canine vaccines by the ministries of health, free delivery of these vaccines, local-level commitment in the planning and execution of the campaigns and effective coordination and supervision of the campaigns by the health services.

At least 70% of the dog population in each community should be vaccinated in areas where canine rabies is endemic. High vaccination coverage (70% or higher) can be attained through strategies consisting of well-designed educational campaigns, intersectoral cooperation, community participation, local commitment in planning and execution, availability of recognized quality vaccine, media support and effective general coordination and supervision of the activities by the health services (*45, 46*).

Rabies vaccination campaigns are generally conducted annually but more frequent campaigns may be required in areas where population birth and death rates are high. All dogs and cats, when presented, should be immunized, regardless of their age, weight or state of health. Given the high birth rates of many populations, particular attention should be paid to ensuring adequate vaccination coverage of puppies (*38*).

In order to apply strategic planning and management, an estimate of the dog population and evaluation of a mass vaccination campaign is required. WHO has produced guidance for estimating dog population size (*46*).

For mass parenteral vaccination campaigns, only inactivated and adjuvanted rabies vaccine should be used.

All personnel handling dogs during vaccination campaigns should receive pre-exposure prophylaxis.

Registration and permanent identification of vaccinated dogs is recommended. However, lack of resources or capacity to permanently identify dogs should not prevent the implementation of a vaccination campaign. The use of temporary coloured tags or plastic collars has proven to be useful in identifying vaccinated dogs and provided motivation for owners to take their pets for vaccination. Identification of dogs is necessary to evaluate the vaccination coverage rate, and to identify unvaccinated dogs for supplementary follow-up measures.

Three basic approaches to mass vaccination campaigns have been adopted, either alone or in combination, to control rabies in canine rabies-endemic areas: house-to-house visits, fixed vaccination posts in well-recognized sites within the community, and mobile teams which set up temporary vaccination posts. Experience has shown that such posts are usually sufficiently attended only from distances of less than 500 m or about 10 minutes' walk. The choice of approach will depend on the specific community and the decision should be taken at the local level. Different strategies may be needed in campaigns designed to control infection in residual foci or to contain new outbreaks.

In some countries, e.g. Sri Lanka, parenteral vaccination campaigns have been combined with the follow-up vaccination of unmarked dogs. Humane killing of unvaccinated dogs after mass vaccination campaigns has been used during campaigns in Malaysia, which succeeded in eliminating dog rabies.

7.3 Supplementary measures: oral vaccination of dogs

Oral vaccination of dogs offers a new approach that may significantly improve dog vaccination coverage (especially of free-roaming and poorly supervised dogs) when applied either exclusively or in combination with parenteral vaccination. As dog accessibility to vaccination by the parenteral route is one of the major obstacles for canine rabies control in many different parts of the world, WHO conducted research on dog populations and dog immunization coverage in various countries in Africa, Latin America and Asia. Acknowledging the limitations of the parenteral route for canine rabies elimination, WHO stimulated studies on oral vaccination of dogs and the development of safer and effective vaccines and baits for such vaccination.

Although the preferential vaccine for dog immunization should be parenteral (inactivated tissue-culture vaccines), oral vaccination should be used whenever there is high population of inaccessible dogs. Further field studies to evaluate economy, efficiency and effectiveness, and demonstrate safety are encouraged. Strategies for vaccine bait distribution must be studied further as new innovations are required for economical distribution.

7.4 Dog population management and animal birth control (ABC) programmes

The Consultation expressed its appreciation of the long-term engagement of WHO to contribute to developing methodologies related to dog ecology and dog population management. Considerable experience has been gained in projects coordinated by WHO in Ecuador, Nepal, Sri Lanka and Tunisia and other ecological studies conducted in South America and Asia. However, data collection needs to be continued in other areas and in countries with different social and ecological conditions.

There is no evidence that removal of dogs alone has ever had a significant impact on dog population densities or the spread of rabies. The population turnover of dogs may be so high that even the highest recorded removal rates (about 15% of the dog population) are easily compensated for by increased survival rates. In addition, dog removal may be unacceptable to local communities. However, the targeted and humane removal of unvaccinated, ownerless dogs may be effective when used as a supplementary measure to mass vaccination.

Several methods to estimate dog population densities based on questionnaire surveys and capture/mark/re-observe studies are available (46). The combination of these two methods allows collection of accurate information on the whole dog population and subpopulations, defined in terms of confinement levels or other parameters. Whereas density estimates based on simple capture/mark/re-observe studies using uniform marking (collars and dyes) are usually adequate in rural areas, more complex study designs involving differential or individual marking are recommended in urban and suburban areas in order to compensate for variations in re-observation probability (1). Questionnaire surveys conducted in the community can be useful where residents recognize the dogs present in their communities.

Three practical methods of dog population management are recognized: movement restriction, habitat control and reproduction control.

Attempts to control dog populations through culling, without alteration of habitat and resource availability, have generally been unsuccessful. Since the 1960s, ABC programmes coupled with rabies vaccination have been advocated as a method to control urban street male and female dog populations and ultimately human rabies in Asia. The rationale is to reduce the dog population turnover as well as the number of dogs susceptible to rabies and limit aspects of male dog behaviour (such as dispersal and fighting) that facilitate the spread of rabies. Culling of dogs during these programmes may be counterproductive as sterilized, vaccinated dogs may be destroyed.

Based on 1990 WHO guidelines (47), ABC programmes have been launched in several countries and the results have been encouraging, with a reported reduction in the size of the street dog population and the number of human rabies cases. However, data are limited and independent evaluation of projects has not yet been undertaken.

7.5 National and international cooperation

Technical cooperation among countries should concern the following closely interrelated elements:

— rapid diagnosis and development of appropriate surveillance for immediate post-exposure prophylaxis in people and disease control in animals;
— antigenic and genetic typing of virus isolates to determine epidemiological patterns and the source of infection in cases occurring before, during and after vaccination campaigns;
— planning, implementing and evaluating national programmes;
— promotion and coordination of control programmes across borders in case of transboundary spread;
— human and animal vaccine procurement through imports or development and transfer of technologies for the production and con-

trol of modern safe and potent vaccines for use in animals and humans;

— provision of training or short-term expertise as required;
— enhanced rabies advocacy to generate public awareness and political commitment for rabies control.

The Consultation recommended that, in this context, four major programme components should be taken into account.

1. The planning and management of community, district, national and regional rabies control programmes.
2. Cooperation with various institutions and the pharmaceutical industry in the provision of vaccines, including promotion of the transfer of technology for rabies vaccine production to developing countries, whenever feasible, and technical cooperation in programme, planning and management to ensure proper vaccine delivery.
3. Promotion of funding by bilateral and multilateral agencies and other donor agencies within the framework of technical cooperation or humanitarian aid.
4. Coordination of international services in collaboration with the Food and Agriculture Organization of the United Nations, the World Organisation for Animal Health (OIE) and nongovernmental organizations such as the World Society for the Protection of Animals (WSPA), and the International Association of Human–Animal Interaction Organizations (IAHAIO).

Designated specialized staff should be posted to WHO regional offices for strengthening the global effort on rabies elimination (45). Governments should be encouraged to establish national focal points, multiyear medium-term plans, and national rabies elimination committees. WHO and WHO collaborating centres and affiliated institutions should cooperate with governments and national institutions to achieve the above goals.

National committees should be actively involved in the management of policies pertaining to rabies control. The public health sector should take the leading role in such committees, with close involvement of other government agencies (those responsible for livestock, veterinary services, local government and natural resources), nongovernmental organizations and private sector agencies.

Efforts should be made to fully incorporate rabies control activities in all levels of the health services, aligning them with other public health programmes such as the Expanded programme on immunization and those for tuberculosis and vector-borne diseases. In this manner, synergies between programmes improve logistical use of human, material and financial resources.

8. Control of rabies in wild animals

In past centuries, rabies was seen predominantly in domestic dogs, though there were reports indicating wildlife involvement. Today, species of the orders Carnivora and Chiroptera are recognized as wildlife reservoirs. The understanding of rabies epidemiology in both orders has significantly changed with the advancement of molecular approaches to virus variant identification.

8.1 Epidemiology and ecology of rabies in carnivore species

8.1.1 *Africa*

Although sporadic cases of rabies in wildlife are documented throughout the African continent, convincing documentation of rabies circulating in populations of wild carnivores exists only for southern Africa. Here, it is useful to distinguish between canid viruses and those transmitted by mongooses. Black-backed and striped jackals (*Canis adustus* and *C. mesomelas*) and bat-eared fox (*Otocyon megalotis*) populations support epizootics of canid rabies viruses. Some rare and endangered African canids are further threatened by spillover from rabies in dogs (documented for the Ethiopian wolf (*C. simensis*) and the African wild dog (*Lycaon pictus*)). A variety of species of the family of mongooses (*Viverridae*) maintain several distinct mongoose rabies virus variants in southern Africa.

Infections with a canid rabies virus have also been the cause of significant mortality in kudus (*Tragelaphus strepsiceros*) in Namibia. It is speculated that there is direct oral transmission of infective saliva from antelope to antelope.

8.1.2 *Asia*

There is very little documentation of wildlife rabies throughout the continent, except for fox rabies in Israel, West Bank and Gaza Strip, some parts of the Arabian Peninsula, and arctic and subarctic areas. Occasional cases in mongooses, jackals (*C. aureus*) and rarely in other wildlife are seen in South and South-East Asia, but these have not been analysed in sufficient detail.

8.1.3 *Europe*

Rabies transmitted by dogs was once widespread in Europe. It started to disappear gradually at the beginning of the 20th century for reasons that are not fully understood. At the beginning of World War II, a new epizootic emerged in eastern Europe. Epidemiological analyses, laboratory studies and modelling suggested that the recent rabies epizootic in western Europe is propagated and maintained by a single species, the red fox (*Vulpes vulpes*). In eastern Europe, introduced raccoon dogs (*Nyctereutes procyonoides*) may be implicated in sustaining the chain of infection. The features of the epizootic expansion in western Europe are well described (*48*). The front moved from Poland to Germany after 1940, reaching France in 1968 and Italy in 1980. Initial outbreaks lasted for about 1 year, usually followed by a period of several months to 2 years without any reported cases and then by oscillating prevalence over many years. These patterns varied from area to area. The first rabies cases recorded in newly affected areas were almost always in foxes. The epizootic front advanced in a wavelike fashion, with a speed of approximately 25–60 km per year. The case density in newly affected areas was usually very high (up to 5 cases/km^2/year). In areas with good surveillance, foxes constituted between 60% and 85% of all diagnosed rabies cases of the initial outbreaks. Large rivers, lakes and high mountain chains functioned as obstacles to the spread. Rivers were usually crossed where bridges were available. Intensive fox destruction campaigns may have stopped the spread in a few privileged locations. The fact that rabies did not invade the Danish peninsula is probably the result of successful fox population reduction across the isthmus. Where rabies alone or in combination with fox control brought fox population density below a certain level, rabies disappeared not only in foxes, but also in all other species (except bats). Analyses of the impact of measures of fox population reduction conducted in France over 10 years (1986–1995) demonstrated that these measures alone cannot control rabies.

The progress of epizootic waves came to a standstill in areas where a proportion of the fox population was immunized through oral vaccination. However, the progression also stopped in northern Italy and in the middle of France without any significant disease control interventions.

Rabies is detected with different frequencies in a wide variety of other species. Such cases are usually in close spatial and temporal proximity to fox rabies cases, but are often separated from other occurrences in the same species. The incidence of rabies in a particular species is dependent upon their susceptibility and the probability of potentially infectious encounters. Animals that inspect or attack a paralysed fox, such as roe deer, cattle and other domestic ruminants, figure more prominently in rabies statistics.

8.1.4 *North America*

The canine rabies epizootic that was predominant historically was brought under control in Canada and in the USA in the middle of the 20th century, and canine rabies is presently being eliminated from Mexico. With the disappearance of canine rabies, wildlife rabies cycles became more and more apparent. In Canada, the most significant vectors are red fox (*V. vulpes*). In the USA, the major hosts are striped skunks (*Mephitis mephitis*) throughout the Plains and in California, and raccoons (*Procyon lotor*) from the Atlantic coast to the Appalachian range. In addition, grey foxes (*Urocyon cinereoargenteus*) are involved (particularly in Texas), several species of skunks (*Spilogale* sp.) are becoming recognized as wildlife vectors in Mexico, and coyotes (*C. latrans*) are spreading a dog rabies virus in Texas. All these species are maintaining one or several distinct variants of the rabies virus.

As in Europe, red fox rabies emerged as a significant epizootic in the middle of the 20th century. In North America, the spread of fox rabies was predominantly north to south into south-eastern Canada and into north-eastern USA. The viruses circulating in European and North American fox populations are distinct, though both are members of the "cosmopolitan branch" in phylogenetic analyses of virus genomes. As in Europe, large areas became free of fox rabies toward the end of the 20th century, in part as a result of oral fox immunization. At the same time as fox rabies expanded its range in the north, a different rabies virus variant emerged in raccoons in the south, in Florida (USA) and spread from there to neighbouring states. The virus was transported with translocated raccoons into the mid-Atlantic area in the 1970s from where it expanded south and north. Spillover into other wildlife and into domestic animals is frequent in all areas.

8.1.5 *South America*

Rabies in terrestrial wildlife has been documented in several areas, though surveillance is generally not intense enough to allow epidemiological analysis. However, a number of molecular studies of the genomes of virus isolates from a variety of species strongly suggest the presence of several distinct terrestrial wildlife reservoirs, such as the marmoset (*Callithrix* sp.) and crab-eating fox (*Cerdocyon* sp.).

8.1.6 *Caribbean islands*

The small Indian mongoose (*Herpestes auropunctatus*) was introduced from South Asia to most Caribbean islands in the second half of the 19th century for rodent control. These animals were recognized as important rabies vectors in the 1950s. For example, mongoose rabies is currently reported in Cuba and the Dominican Republic.

8.1.7 *Eurasian and American arctic and subarctic regions*

Arctic foxes (*Alopex lagopus*) and domestic dogs, along with red foxes, appear to participate in the propagation of arctic rabies or "polar madness", though the epidemiology is not well understood in these thinly populated areas with incomplete surveillance. It has been speculated that these "arctic reservoirs" were the origin of the red fox rabies epizootics in North America and Europe in the second half of the 20th century.

8.2 Rabies in bats

Lyssaviruses have been detected in bats in several different continents and bats have been identified as vectors for six of the seven *Lyssavirus* genotypes characterized so far (see section 2.2). Chiroptera have life-history traits that are quite different from those of carnivore rabies hosts: they are small, long lived, have low intrinsic population growth rates and and different bat species occupy a variety of well-defined ecological niches. The properties of lyssaviruses adapted to bats must therefore be different from those causing Carnivora rabies. This statement remains a hypothesis because the population biology and epidemiology of bat rabies are insufficiently explored.

8.2.1 *Lyssaviruses in Africa, Australia and Eurasia*

The African bat lyssavirus isolates are of genotypes 2 and 4, while those from bats in Europe have been identified as genotypes 5 and 6.

Lagos bat virus (LBV) is a virus (genotype 2) of large African fruit bats (*Megachiroptera*). It was originally isolated from *Eidolon helvum* in Nigeria in 1956, then was later isolated from other bat species in the Central African Republic, Senegal and South Africa. An epizootic causing significant mortality in *Epomophorus* bats was observed in Natal, South Africa, from where the virus is still occasionally isolated. No human cases have been confirmed to date.

Duvenhage virus (DUVV) (genotype 4) was first isolated in 1970 from a person who died of rabies encephalitis, 5 weeks after being bitten by an insectivorous bat in Transvaal, South Africa. Later the virus was also found in two insectivorous bats, one in South Africa and one in Zimbabwe.

In Europe unexplained sporadic cases of rabies were diagnosed in bats for over the last 50 years. In 1985, a bat biologist died of rabies in Finland. At the same time epizootics in serotine bats (*Eptesicus serotinus*) were recorded in other parts of northern Europe, mostly in Denmark and the Netherlands. Today, two groups of bat viruses are recognized in Europe: those originating from serotine bats are identified as EBLV-1 (genotype 5), while those from rare isolates from *Myotis* bats (*M. dasycneme* and *M. daubentonii*) are named EBLV-2 (genotype 6). In total, four human rabies cases transmitted by bats have been confirmed in Europe; two in the Russian Federation (1977 and 1985), one in Finland (1985) and the most recent in Scotland (2002).

In 1996, a new lyssavirus, ABLV (genotype 7) was isolated from fruit-eating bats (flying foxes, *Pteropus alecto*) on the eastern coast of Australia, a country considered to be rabies free since 1867. A subtype of this genotype was also isolated from insectivorous bats. Two human rabies deaths caused by the ABLV have been confirmed in Australia.

The distribution of the insectivorous bat species recognized as hosts of lyssaviruses in Europe extends into Asia. There is very little doubt that EBLV-related viruses will be found in Asia. Similarly, it is not hard to imagine that the lyssaviruses found in bats in Australia have their counterparts in southern Asia. No such isolates have been recovered to date.

8.2.2 *Rabies in insectivorous bats in the Americas*

To date, New World bat rabies viruses have all been categorized as genotype 1. In the Americas a large number of genetically and antigenically distinct genotype 1 variants circulate in different bat species. Several variants occur in a single species, and the geographical distribution of variants is overlapping. Spillover to terrestrial animals is observed frequently. Though the incidence of human rabies is low in temperate North America, approximately half of the cases are caused by infections with bat rabies viruses, most frequently with a virus that is associated with silverhaired bats (*Lasionycteris noctivagans*) and eastern pipistrelle bats (*Pipistrellus subflavus*).

8.2.3 *Vampire bat rabies*

Vampire bat rabies is a major public health problem in subtropical and tropical areas of the Americas, including the Caribbean. A genotype 1 virus related to the other American bat viruses is maintained in haematophagous bats, mainly by *Desmodus rotundus*. It is frequently transmitted to domestic animals and humans. Vampire bat-transmitted bovine paralytic rabies has a significant economic impact on livestock industries.

8.3 Rabies in rodents

Examination of tens of thousands of wild and synanthropic rodents in endemic rabies areas in North America and Europe has revealed only rare instances of rodent rabies infection, indicating that these animals do not serve as reservoirs of the disease.

8.4 Wildlife species of special concern

Rabies has emerged as a disease of conservation concern following rabies outbreaks in highly endangered populations of Ethiopian wolves (*C. simensis*) in the Bale Mountains National Park, in African wild dogs (*Lycaon pictus*) in eastern and southern Africa, and in Blanford's fox (*Vulpes cana*) in Israel. Ethiopian wolves and African wild dogs are among the world's most endangered carnivore species and transmission of rabies from more abundant reservoir hosts (such as domestic dogs) is considered an extinction threat for several populations.

Rabies has been recorded in wolves everywhere in the northern hemisphere where rabies in wolves and other wildlife co-occur. Rabies in wolves is often experienced as a dramatic event, particularly if people are involved. Wolves are susceptible to the disease and readily succumb to it. Once a pack member is infected, the disease can decimate the pack because of its highly social nature, with regular contact between the animals. However, because of the highly territorial nature of wolves, it is not common for the disease to spread from one pack to another. At least in North America, wolves do not contribute significantly to the maintenance of rabies in the wild. All cases investigated carried viruses with the exact genetic make-up as those found in fox rabies cases in their vicinity. Wolf populations may also not have the densities and dynamics to support epizootics independent of other wildlife.

At the beginning of the 20th century, the raccoon dog (*Nyctereutes procyonoides*) was introduced from Asia into the western part of the former Soviet Union. Since this time, this highly opportunistic species has invaded large regions in north-eastern Europe, with a tendency to spread westwards. In some regions in eastern Europe, the raccoon dog established population densities higher than those of the fox. In some Baltic countries, the number of cases in raccoon dogs has recently exceeded that of foxes. It is not clear yet whether raccoon dogs maintain a distinct epidemiological cycle.

8.5 Elimination of rabies in wild Carnivora

8.5.1 *Reduction of animal populations*

Rabies transmission within animal populations is density dependent. The objective of wildlife culling is to lower population densities below the threshold necessary to maintain the disease. Culling techniques include hunting, trapping, poisoning and den gassing. Studies on the effect of culling reservoir species on the control of rabies show that there are only very few examples where such methods alone have either eliminated the disease or have prevented its spread to previously uninfected areas. The resilience of these Carnivora to persecution, their high reproductive potential, together with the capacity of the environment to provide food, water and shelter, most often render population control efforts futile. Humane and ecological aspects should be considered before engaging in large-scale culling campaigns.

A more promising approach would be to combine population reduction with immunization, as has been successfully applied in Canada in 1999 to stop the advancing raccoon rabies epizootic.

8.5.2 *Wildlife immunization*

The idea that mass immunization of the principal wildlife hosts might be more effective than culling emerged independently in North America and Europe. Europeans were certainly keen to adopt more humane rabies control techniques and to abandon the cruel methods of the 1960s and 1970s. Attempts in Europe to trap wild carnivores and to release them after parenteral vaccination were rapidly abandoned, though such trap–vaccinate–release procedures are still used with apparent success in some areas of Canada. It appears more promising to lure the wild mammal into vaccinating itself. This is possible when oral vaccines are included in baits targeted at the principal host species. In the early 1960s, George Baer found that foxes in the USA could be immunized by oral application of the live attenuated ERA virus. The discovery, which did not gather much attention until it was presented at a WHO-sponsored conference held in Europe in 1970, became more accessibly published in 1971. The later development of other oral rabies vaccines brought with it the new dimensions of industry involvement, with property rights and patents, which have both facilitated and constrained research on oral vaccines.

In 1978, the late Franz Steck, leader of a Swiss rabies research team, concluded that the time was right for a first field application. This conclusion was reached only after extensive data had been obtained from numerous laboratory and field studies on efficacy and safety. Switzerland was joined 5 years later by Germany, by Italy in 1984 and by other European countries after 1985. The first field trials in the Swiss Rhone Valley were possible because of the informed courage of all the key players, which included scientists and government officials. This represented a significant fait accompli that later facilitated similar decisions in other European countries, and in Canada and the USA. The vaccines presently applied in the field include a variety of derivatives of ERA and VRG (see section 5.2).

Oral rabies vaccination programmes should result in sufficient herd immunity to reduce transmission (i.e. the effective reproductive rate of the disease, R_0, falls below 1). The level of herd immunity that is required is controversial; it no doubt varies in accordance with the disease transmission dynamics in particular species and populations.

Vaccine efficacy is determined in laboratory experiments, typically by following guidelines from international organizations (*33, 34*) and national legislation, though the target population in the field, affected by all kinds of immunocompromising conditions, may not be as responsive as animals tested in the laboratory. Baits must be designed to release the vaccine onto a susceptible target tissue of the bait consumer (*49*). A vaccine that is inactivated by the degrading stomach environment must be delivered into either the oral cavity to infect cells in the oropharyngeal mucosa or tonsils, or the baits (or bait components) have to protect it from passage through the stomach and release it into the small intestine. Vaccine efficacy and stability and effective vaccine release from the bait control the percentage of bait consumers that become immunized. Spatial and temporal bait distribution routines that make baits available to potential consumers influence the proportion of the target population that consumes them within the time-limits of vaccine degradation. Only a fraction of all baits deposited during a baiting campaign are picked up by the target species. How many are removed by competitors depends on bait specificity; however, even a very specific bait may not be attractive enough to ensure sufficient bait uptake. Attractiveness of a bait changes from habitat to habitat, as each offers to foragers a different range of food choices. Our understanding of target species as "optimal foragers" suggests that a particular bait type may be well suited for certain local and seasonal conditions only. In Europe, oral vaccination campaigns are generally conducted on a biannual basis, in spring and in autumn, using fixed-wing aircrafts or helicopters for bait delivery. Manual distribution is successful in suburban areas as a complement to aerial distribution.

To date, seven European countries are reported by OIE to be free of terrestrial rabies as a result of successful oral vaccination programmes (*50*): Finland and the Netherlands since 1991, Italy since 1997, Switzerland since 1998, France since 2000, and Belgium and Luxembourg since 2001.

8.5.3 *Planning, implementation and evaluation of oral vaccination programmes*

Oral immunization of wild animals has become the essential tool of programmes for the control and elimination of rabies where a wildlife reservoir exists. Basic requirements for planning, implementing and evaluating large-scale field trials for the oral immunization of wild animals have been elaborated by WHO (*49*) and the European Commission (*50*).

Vaccine and bait selection
Vaccine selection: vaccine efficacy in the target species needs to be considered. Preference should be given to vaccines with reduced (non-rabies related) pathogenicity, such as recombinant vaccines (VRG) or a highly attenuated live virus strain (SAG2), over more pathogenic attenuated live viruses for oral immunization of wildlife and dogs.

Programmes for the control of wildlife rabies should take into consideration both target and non-target species of wildlife populations, in order to select the most effective baiting methodology available. Epidemiological data based on reliable surveillance and laboratory studies of rabies cases in target and non-target species must be available before field trials are initiated. Estimates of target population size should be obtained as well as the estimation of bait biomarker background in the target species before vaccination. It is also recommended that possible effects on non-target species, particularly on endangered species, be evaluated. For dealing with possible or perceived adverse events of recombinant vaccines, such as reassortment with similar animal viruses circulating in nature, it is advisable that the prevalence of agents related to the vector virus(es) in target and non-target species populations as well as their propagation in previously unrecognized host(s) be monitored.

Project planning
Project planning must precede the distribution of baits, and related administrative activities will vary in structure and detail depending

upon political and other variables. Planning and organization are vital to the success of the project. The project should be based on a comprehensive plan that justifies it, describes the objectives, technical and organizational details, budgetary requirements, and defines the responsibilities of the collaborating institutions. A project proposal must also include background information on the geographical area to be covered using oral rabies vaccination, estimated costs and benefits of the project, timing, safety considerations, methods of post-baiting evaluation and relevant data on the target population. The project should also include details of the short- and long-term vaccination policy that will be conducted at country level. The proposal should be distributed to the institutions concerned well in advance for consideration and evaluation. Upon request, WHO may help in providing the necessary expertise.

If several geographical locations are available for the implementation of field trials, priority should be given to those surrounded by natural barriers and/or where community cooperation and logistic support can be relied upon. The rabies situation in neighbouring areas should also be taken into account. The selected areas should be readily accessible to government veterinary and medical services. To guarantee effective control of rabies, the size of the vaccinated area should reflect the ecological and epidemiological attributes of the specific situation, such as the home range, movement patterns of wildlife populations and geographical characteristics of the area.

Implementation
Implementation of oral wildlife immunization projects necessitates logistics that ensure bait and vaccine integrity, and processes that allow the distribution of adequate numbers of baits to evenly cover large areas. In addition the following may be required:

— community participation. This should be encouraged through information, promotion campaigns and, in some instances, training for baiting and disease surveillance;
— awareness of the campaign among medical and veterinary practitioners, so that they can take appropriate measures in case of accidental exposure to the vaccine. A medical/veterinary advisory group should be established;
— sampling of specimens under appropriate conditions. Trained personnel and laboratory facilities should be available to carry out the tests for campaign evaluation as well as the estimation of bait biomarkers and serological determination in the target species, along with the continuation of rabies surveillance;
— assignment of specialists to investigate the epidemiological situa-

tion in both humans and animals before, during, and after the implementation of the project, and to report to the responsible authorities on a regular basis. After each campaign, evaluation of results is of utmost importance in order to adapt future strategies.

Evaluation of oral vaccination programmes
Most field trials using oral vaccination employ several methods of evaluation: testing for the occurrence of biomarkers (usually tetracycline), which is incorporated into the bait, in the target species; examining sera from the target species for rabies antibodies; and analysing the prevalence of rabies before, during and after the programme.

Rabies surveillance plays an important part in the planning, implementation and evaluation of rabies control programmes. Before oral vaccination programmes are carried out, rabies surveillance is usually sufficient. Generally, surveillance is also sufficient during vaccination campaigns, particularly where hunters and wildlife services are engaged in sampling of field animals and active sampling is supported by granting appropriate incentives to hunters and trappers. However, experience has shown that the intensity of surveillance activities decreases as successive cycles of oral vaccination campaigns are completed. Adequate surveillance is most important during this phase; the absence of rabies requires verification, and residual foci of rabies must be detected rapidly. It is important to collect animal samples, particularly from animals that are ill or found dead to monitor the impact of vaccination.

For the monitoring of the efficacy of oral vaccination programmes (biomarker detection, serological testing and rabies incidence) a minimum of four target animals per $100\,km^2$ should be investigated annually.

The Consultation stressed the need for reinforced rabies surveillance in oral vaccination areas and requests governments to consider and adopt the above guidelines.

To promote active rabies surveillance in areas where oral vaccination campaigns have been successful, procedures for international certification of the rabies-free status should be established.

International cooperation in oral vaccination programmes
International cooperation in border areas is essential at all levels to achieve effective control programmes. Neighbouring countries should carefully coordinate their activities along common borders. If field trials reach a country border, local administrative staff from both countries should coordinate their efforts. WHO may be helpful in

assisting in the coordination of rabies vaccination programmes involving borders between countries.

Oral rabies vaccination generates new epidemiological and ecological concerns within and beyond national borders. For this reason, planning, implementation and evaluation of campaigns should be coordinated at country as well as international levels. Preliminary contacts should be made with neighbouring countries when oral vaccination policy is decided; these contacts should be maintained through regular regional meetings till the elimination of the disease. The assistance of WHO collaborating centres and of other international organizations is recommended.

8.6 Bat rabies control

Vampire bat-transmitted paralytic rabies of cattle can be controlled by vaccination of cattle. The only presently available approach to control in the vector species is culling. This can be achieved by administration of anticoagulant to vampire bats, either by direct application of the substance on the backs of captured bats or by the intramuscular injection of warfarin to cattle. Non-specific methods that indiscriminately destroy haematophagous, frugivorous, nectarivorous and insectivorous bat species must be avoided.

Approaches to control the transmission of insectivorous bat rabies to people should include education of the public to avoid potentially infectious contact with bats, to seek proper treatment after exposure and to prevent bats from establishing colonies in certain sensitive buildings (e.g. hospitals and schools). Preventive immunization of populations living in highly endemic areas should be considered.

8.7 Other public health measures

It is recommended to provide education to avoid direct contact with wildlife in general, and with abnormally behaving and sick animals in particular. Any person bitten by a wild animal, including bats, must seek medical attention. The culling of insectivorous bat species is not warranted and should be avoided as much as possible because of the protected status of these bats in most countries. Translocation of wildlife for any purpose, except conservation, should be banned or strongly discouraged.

---

[1] To be decided by the relevant regional or international authority.
[2] Suspect cases may need to be defined, e.g. as individuals of susceptible species showing encephalitis-like symptoms or dying of an unknown cause.

9. Rabies-free and provisionally rabies-free countries or areas

A rabies-free country or area — for the purpose of assisting public health authorities in assessing the risk of rabies associated with contact with animals and the need for rabies post-exposure prophylaxis — is defined as one in which:

— no case of indigenously acquired infection by a lyssavirus has been confirmed in humans or any animal species, including bats, at any time during the previous 2 years; and
— an adequate surveillance system is in operation. The system should include or be able to have easy access to one rabies laboratory using WHO-recommended techniques for rabies diagnosis, which tests a minimum number[1] of samples from suspect[2] cases belonging to the major susceptible domestic and wild animal species present in the country and reports only negative results. National public health and veterinary authorities in collaboration with relevant international entities should define the appropriate number of samples to be tested from the different susceptible wild and domestic species. National authorities should ensure that the samples are collected homogenously throughout the country and on a regular basis during the year. Priority has to be given to the examination of animals showing abnormal behaviour, suspected of being rabid, and those found dead such as road kills. For domestic animals, in particular dogs and cats, the number of samples to be tested should be between 0.01% and 0.02% of the estimated population. Serology for wild animals should be considered as an indicator of the rabies situation; and
— an effective import policy is implemented, i.e. measures to prevent the importation of rabies, especially those proposed in section 10.2, are in place.

Additional measures may also be in place, such as vaccination of dogs and other pets, and animal population management activities.

A provisionally rabies-free country or area is either:

— historically free of rabies and an adequate rabies surveillance system and an effective import policy have been put into place to confirm and ensure maintenance of the rabies-free status; or
— an area of a rabies-infected country where a successful animal rabies elimination programme is continuing and where an adequate rabies surveillance system and an effective import policy have been put into place to confirm the rabies-free status.

A provisionally rabies-free area becomes rabies free when it fulfils all the conditions above.

10. International transfer of animals

For the purpose of this report, the terms companion animals and pets refer to dogs and cats; in the case of European Union regulations, they also include ferrets. Historically, most countries free of rabies (except in bats) had in place a very strict quarantine system for all domestic and wild animals, which served as a strong deterrent for most people to travel with their pets. In 1993, New Caledonia implemented a system modifying quarantine laws for cats and dogs, based on a valid anti-rabies vaccination certificate in addition to the results of a serological test and a certificate of good health. Similar measures have now been adopted by other countries. Currently, the regulations for importing companion animals into rabies-free countries or areas vary according to national government regulations. For example, there are differences in the number of serological tests required, the interval between rabies vaccination and serological testing, as well as between serological testing and the allowed entry date, and the requirement of additional quarantine time upon arrival. These requirements should not preclude the application of more stringent measures by government authorities.

10.1 International transport of companion animals from rabies-infected countries or areas to rabies-free countries or areas

Each rabies-free country, when establishing its own guidelines (51) and requirements, should take into consideration the following:

— all pets should have an international veterinary certificate and be identifiable by means of a microchip. Tattoos will be accepted until 2008 in some European countries and in other countries, but as they can become unreadable with time, they should be discouraged. In some countries and regions such as Europe, USA, New Zealand and the West Indies, microchips must comply with Standards 11784/Annex A of 11785 (International Organization for Standardization). If the microchip cannot be read by a standard reader, the owner should supply the necessary equipment to allow accurate identification of the animal;

— all pets should be vaccinated with an inactivated vaccine produced in cell culture, containing a minimum of one antigenic unit per dose or, wherever they are licensed, with a recombinant vaccine. The animal should not be younger than 3 months (or 2 months in the case of recombinant vaccines for cats). Following primary vaccination, older animals should then receive a second vaccination 1 year later, followed by boosters every 1 to 3 years, depending on the manufacturer's recommendations and regulations in each country. In the case of primary vaccination, entry into a rabies-free country cannot take place before 6 months and after 12 months following vaccination. In the case of a booster vaccination, the last vaccination must be within 12 months of the date of entry.

— all pets entering a rabies-free country or area should be tested at least once and should have a minimum rabies-neutralizing antibody titre of 0.5 IU/ml a minimum of 90 days and a maximum of 24 months from vaccination to entry into the country or area. For this purpose, two tests are recommended by OIE (18): the RFFIT or FAVN test (52, 53). Rabies-free countries should provide a list of approved laboratories which are officially recognized to perform one of the approved tests;

— companion animals not complying with all of these requirements should be refused entry or be subjected to a strict quarantine of 6 months, as determined by the regulations of individual rabies-free countries or areas.

10.2 International transport of companion animals between rabies-free countries or areas

Transport of companion animals with documented origin between rabies-free countries or areas that benefit from an insular situation, such as between the United Kingdom and Ireland, or Hawaii and Australia, should be unrestricted, provided that this meets all national requirements.

10.3 Special exemption for guide dogs for people with disabilities and other service dogs

Certified guide dogs for people with disabilities and other service dogs (e.g. military and search dogs) already present in rabies-free countries should be permitted to accompany their owners into rabies-infected countries if the dogs are vaccinated with a cell-culture vaccine fulfilling WHO and OIE requirements and demonstrated to have adequate virus-neutralizing antibody titre, using one of the two methods recommended by OIE (18). These dogs must be identifiable by means of a microchip. Provided that the owners confirm that they were kept confined, on a leash or under permanent visual supervision while abroad in a rabies-infected country, the dogs should be allowed to remain outside the country for a maximum of 6 months without any requirements for re-entry other than reconfirmation of the antibody titre.

10.4 International transport of livestock, zoo, research and show animals from rabies-infected countries or areas to rabies-free countries or areas

Countries that are free from rabies should either prohibit the importation of certain species of mammals, in particular Carnivora and Chiroptera, or permit their entry only under licence, subject to quarantine in premises and under conditions approved by the government veterinary service. Entry may be permitted for limited periods or for life. The use of animals for exhibits or for experiments should be permitted only after quarantine for 4 months.

In view of the increase in the number or reported rabies cases in wild animals acquired as pets, national authorities should control the trade in such animals because of this potential source of human exposure. The keeping of such animals as pets should be discouraged. Adequate quarantine measures should be adopted for at least 4 months, combined with vaccination with inactivated vaccines.

For other species not covered in this section, refer to the OIE *Terrestrial animal health code (51)*.

10.5 International transport of any animal from rabies-free to rabies-infected countries or areas or between rabies-infected countries or areas

Such animals should meet all international recommendations. If transported from rabies-free to rabies-infected countries they should be vaccinated at least 2 weeks prior to embarkation. If transported between two rabies-infected countries they should be vaccinated at least 2 weeks before embarkation or vaccinated on arrival in the country of destination.

11. Exchange of information

11.1 Collection of epidemiological data

The WHO World Survey of Rabies has been enhanced by a computerized data management system, Rabnet, which has collected rabies data electronically since the early 1990s. It became accessible through the Internet for data consultation and online data entry in 2000. In 2003, Rabnet2 was launched (see Annex 6):[1] it retains the same concept as the former Rabnet, and now provides additional features such

---

[1] http://www.who.int/rabies/rabnet

as interactive maps of rabies data at global and country levels. It is anticipated that in the near future, the interactive maps will reflect data at district and even community levels. It also provides a resource library containing ready-made maps and lyssavirus-related documents; it also coordinates and provides details of the WHO collaborating centres for rabies. Rabies data can be linked to a broad range of country-specific indicators (population, education and health services) to provide a more comprehensive picture of the rabies situation of a given country at different levels.

The most important part of this new system is the online data questionnaire. The questionnaire has been simplified: it streamlines the process of entering and validating data. Hard copies of the questionnaire are still distributed to national rabies programme managers and are used as back-up especially if remote data entry is difficult or impossible.

Rabnet data management and processing have been improved to deliver better charts, graphs and maps and decrease the time required for entering data into the system. This database has been extremely helpful in analysing global trends of the disease as well as regional changes, especially in regions where surveillance systems are weak or lacking (3). In 2002, WHO created a rabies web site[1] that provides information on rabies epidemiology worldwide, the disease in humans and animals, human and animal vaccines, and post-exposure prophylaxis. It also includes portable document format versions of selected WHO reports on rabies published during the past 15 years.

11.2 Regional activities for rabies information exchange

Several regional initiatives and venues for information sharing have developed rapidly and continued to flourish in the last decade. The initiatives are of great value for human and animal rabies surveillance for everyone working towards rabies control and eventual elimination. National authorities should be aware of these surveillance activities and venues for information sharing on rabies provided by international and regional organizations and institutions.

11.2.1 *Africa*

The Southern and Eastern Africa Rabies Group has organized seven regional meetings between 1992 and 2003 and the proceedings have been published (54–60). These meetings have consistently aimed at establishing the true burden of rabies in Africa and improving the diagnosis, control and prevention programmes.

---

[1] http://www.who.int/rabies

11.2.2 *Asia*

International symposia on rabies control in Asia have been convened four times between 1988 and 2001 (*38, 61–63*). The proceedings of these meetings have been an important tool for information exchange and technical updating for Asian national control programme officers and international experts. The WHO Regional Office for South-East Asia convened one intercountry meeting in 1998 to develop a regional strategy for rabies elimination; WHO headquarters organized an international consultation in 2001 on prevention and control of rabies in the South-East Asia Region (*45*) and a third intercountry meeting on rabies is proposed for 2005. In 2001, the fourth international symposium on rabies control in Asia was convened by WHO, in collaboration with the Fondation Marcel Mérieux, in Hanoi, Viet Nam, for the purpose of addressing the technical, scientific and operational aspects of the problem in Asia (*38*). The Steering Committee for Rabies Control in Asia led by WHO was established to focus on four aspects namely: (a) surveillance and data collection; (b) national and regional collaboration; (c) research and development; and (d) advocacy. The Steering Committee has met five times from December 2001–December 2003 and will be reconvened on an annual basis from 2005.

11.2.3 *Americas*

The Regional Information System for Epidemiologic Surveillance of Rabies in the Americas (SIRVERA) of PAHO/WHO Regional Office for the Americas produces an annual report on rabies from data provided by the countries. Every 2 years PAHO convenes the Meeting of the Directors of the National Rabies Programme (REDIPRA) where information on rabies and the strategies for rabies control are discussed and updated. The conclusions and recommendations of the REDIPRA are submitted to the ministers of health and ministers of agriculture of the PAHO Member countries during the Inter-American Meeting at the Ministerial Level on Health and Agriculture (RIMSA). The International Conference of Rabies in the Americas has been organized annually to review and discuss the state of the art of rabies research and control in the region. The 15th meeting was held in the Dominican Republic in October 2004.

11.2.4 *Europe*

The WHO Collaborating Centre for Rabies Surveillance and Research, Friedrich Loeffler Institute in Wusterhausen, Germany, has produced the *Rabies Bulletin Europe* since 1977. The bulletin describes the reported rabies cases in Europe by quarter. Online

---

[1] http://www.who-rabies-bulletin.org

publishing of the bulletin started in 1999.[1] Since 2003, the bulletin has contained data from western, central and eastern European countries, including the Russian Federation and some of the Newly Independent States. The WHO Collaborating Centre for Research and Management in Zoonoses Control, Malzéville, France and the WHO Collaborating Centre for Rabies Surveillance and Research, Wusterhausen, Germany, have organized 10 meetings since 1985 on rabies control in central and eastern European countries. The proceedings and recommendations of these meetings have been published. The latest was the WHO meeting on rabies control in middle and east European countries, in Kosice, Slovakia, in September 2002 (*64*).

11.2.5 *Mediterranean*

The WHO Mediterranean Zoonoses Control Center regularly produces its *Information Circular* with special issues on human and animal rabies.

11.3 Seminars, group training and fellowships

Regional and interregional seminars and training courses in the planning and management of zoonoses control programmes, supported by WHO, its regional offices and their specialized centres, have continued to include rabies.

Training workshops and fellowships concerning public health and veterinary aspects of rabies control and prevention have been provided to individuals. A number of national and regional workshops on the clinical management of patients potentially exposed to rabies have also been supported by WHO. Some WHO-supported training activities also include zoonoses field control operations, diagnosis, surveillance, control and research projects, with special attention to rabies, to improve the participants' knowledge of advances in rabies control. These activities promote the adoption of harmonized and improved methods of animal rabies control, aimed ultimately at preventing human disease.

12. Research considerations for the 21st century

12.1 Basic research

12.1.1 *Diagnostics*

The direct FA technique has served as the cornerstone of rabies diagnosis for the past half century. Nevertheless, detailed standard operating procedures and appropriate equipment and reagents for rabies diagnosis are often lacking globally and only few confirmatory tests are performed in humans and animals in some regions. Improved tests for rapid and economical diagnosis, with no loss in sensitivity or specificity, would be welcome. Similarly, for molecular methods, the identification of more universal primers, real-time reverse transcription-PCR and nested PCR assays, a greater focus upon other viral genes besides N and G, and improved sequencing protocols are needed, especially for developing countries where lyssavirus diversity is underappreciated.

12.1.2 *Molecular, genetic and epidemiological characterization of new isolates*

New isolates are being reported more frequently from different parts of the world. Scientists participating in the discovery of new lyssaviruses should be encouraged to act promptly to characterize these isolates. Antigenic, genetic and epidemiological methods have been developed and many lyssavirus sequences are now available in public databases for comparison with new isolates and for phylogenetic analysis. In addition, molecular tools, including restriction fragment length polymorphism and genotype-specific primers, have been developed for rapid screening and classification of new isolates. It is of particular importance to verify if rabies biologicals, such as vaccines and antibodies, protect against newly isolated viruses.

12.1.3 *Biologicals*

After the advent of cell-culture-based vaccines in the 1970s, no major advances have occurred in the development of new human rabies biologicals, as far as commercial realization is concerned. Of several options for future paradigm shifts, the technology available via reverse genetics opens powerful arenas to use negative-stranded RNA viruses as cloning and expression vectors. Additionally, newer, safer and more effective recombinant viruses, for example focused upon adenoviruses, as well as DNA and plant-based vaccines, should continue to receive greater attention. In all cases, the use of genetically engineered rabies vaccines should comply with national and international biosafety guidelines. Assuming continued emergence of new lyssaviruses, especially in bats, the need of a broader protection spectrum of rabies vaccines is needed. For example, DNA vaccines with plasmids expressing chimeric G protein(s) made from the fusion of two halves (part) of G originating from different genotypes have induced in mice antibodies with a wider spectrum of neutralization against various lyssaviruses. These chimeric G proteins could be used to prepare anti-lyssavirus vaccines. In addition, insertion of foreign epitopes/antigens within the lyssavirus G protein was also demonstrated in mice and offers perspectives to prepare a multivalent vaccine (65–67). Activation of innate immune responses by novel vaccine carriers and adjuvants and their protection when used for post-exposure prophylaxis should be further elucidated.

The opportunity to combine basic rabies parenteral or oral vaccination with concomitant immunocontraception for dogs and other carnivores is also of value. Similarly, pragmatic methods other than population reduction for the control of rabies in vampire bats should be investigated.

Besides vaccines, rabies immunoglobulin is a critical part of human rabies post-exposure prophylaxis, particularly after severe and multiple bites to the face by rabid carnivores. In addition to standard laboratory potency tests that determine the relative concentration of rabies virus neutralizing antibodies per unit volume, some measure of expected efficacy is desirable. Reproducible animal models should be developed to assess the effectiveness of various immunoglobsulins after rabies virus infection. The in vivo half-life of antibody preparations in relevant target tissues should be established for new immunoglobulin preparations. Levels of antibodies needed for successful passive immunization and their duration should be established. Immunoglobulin preparations that may have to be given repeatedly need to be tested for potential interference with active immunization. Animal models may be useful to generate data needed for the assessment of suitable immunoglobulins or alternatives, such as monoclonal antibodies, in modern rabies prophylaxis.

The current NIH test for vaccine potency is fraught with difficulties, and more appropriate methods to assess the relative antigenic content are desirable.

12.1.4 *Treatment*

At least five patients that had all received either pre- or post-exposure prophylaxis developed clinical signs of rabies and subsequently recovered. In 2004, a teenager in Wisconsin, USA, bitten by a bat became the first person to recover from the disease after experimental therapy that included a drug-induced coma, with no use of rabies biologicals. In keeping with recent communications on the palliative treatment of human rabies victims, new research on antiviral drugs, focused on negative-stranded RNA viruses, should be supported. Current research on short interfering RNA should be expanded to include the lyssaviruses.

Combined with realistic animal models, a holistic approach should entail rapid intra vitam diagnostics, basic patient care, vaccination, administration of immunoglobulins, cytokines, etc. Insights gleaned from pathobiological studies can be used in the design of additional approaches in the future.

12.1.5 *Epidemiology*

Recent observations suggest that bats are important lyssavirus reservoirs, and the virus variants associated with Chiroptera may occasionally spill over into other mammals, with the potential for adaptation and establishment. It is particularly disturbing that there is sometimes no evidence of direct exposure in human cases of infection associated with bats. New research should focus on the epidemiology of bat lyssaviruses and potential pathogenic mechanisms. No recent comprehensive studies exist using relevant hosts and viruses, or alternative routes and unusual settings.

12.1.6 *Pathobiology*

Lyssaviruses naturally infect neurones resulting in dysfunction and death. Further fundamental studies are required to understand the molecular basis of rabies pathobiology in neurones and other relevant tissues. The diversity of lyssavirus genotypes offers opportunities to address these questions through their differential pathogenicity in cell and animal models.

Recently, organs (including kidneys and liver) were transplanted from a misdiagnosed patient to other humans and caused rabies. The wide distribution of virus throughout the body may compel us to revise our views about rabies transmission. Rather than discourage organ donation or transplantation, such scenarios should be viewed as important opportunities to review current practices to determine if there are ways to enhance the safety of transplant procedures without having an impact on organ supply, as well as to raise questions about basic rabies pathogenesis. For example, the likely mechanism of infection during transplantation remains unclear. Similarly, the effects of patient immune suppression on disease development are not predictable. Prevention and rapid screening for recognition of transplant-transmitted infections may be improved in various ways, including the development of appropriate animal models to study the process of overall pathobiology.

There is a need to investigate in experimental animals at what stage of infection the virus is present in organs other than the CNS. Clinicians treating human rabies cases should be encouraged to obtain, in the course of the disease, samples of secretions, blood and other body fluids and tissues for testing for the presence of rabies virus.

New vaccines, immunoglobulins, cytokines and antivirals should be used in an experimental setting in preparation for any future suspected cases that may arise if an organ recipient has received an implant from a donor who was later found by screening or diagnostic follow-up to have been infected with rabies virus.

12.2 Operational research for canine rabies control

Operational research should be conducted to remove or alleviate the main constraints and obstacles to canine rabies control programmes, which, as outlined below, include a lack of visibility, coordination, infrastructure, dog population management and community awareness.

12.2.1 *Rabies: a priority in national health policy*

In rabies-endemic countries with a high number of rabies deaths per 100 000 inhabitants, ways and means to bring rabies to the priority level it deserves as part of the national health policy should be identified. Rabies should be listed as an important health problem in countries with high reported or estimated numbers of human rabies deaths and providing large number of post-exposure prophylaxis annually.

12.2.2 *Coordinated national rabies programme*

In most countries, several ministries deal with rabies. Generally the ministry of health is responsible for the prevention of rabies in humans and the ministry of agriculture is in charge of rabies control in animals. The ministry of local government and/or the ministries of commerce, industry or science and technologies are involved in rabies vaccine production and imports, dog population management and dog immunization. NGOs and animal rights and welfare groups also have a stake in rabies control and often these groups and organizations act independently and in tandem. The interaction and collaboration between the veterinary and public health departments is minimal or non-existent at all levels in most countries, resulting in unproductive use of resources. A central coordinating body or mechanism should be established to ensure that the efforts for rabies control are cohesive and give satisfactory results.

12.2.3 *Supportive laws and regulations*

Most countries have laws and regulations regarding stray animals, animal transportation and ownership of pets, including registration and vaccination requirements. However, in many of those affected by endemic dog rabies, these laws and regulations are not complied with, because they are unenforceable under the prevalent cultural, social and economic constraints. Alternative approaches, such as the implementation of "soft" population control projects (such as ABC) and education on proper health behaviour, responsible dog ownership and proper rubbish disposal, should be studied and, where feasible, their implementation promoted. The need for laws and regulations for such alternative programmes should be considered in the future. Clearly, stray dog removal and other accompanying measures described above must be carried out wherever these measures are effective.

12.2.4 *Infrastructure and capacity*

The majority of rabies-endemic countries are some of the least developed, riddled with problems of inadequate health infrastructure, inadequate manpower, limited access to populations, few resources for health, and with the majority of people caught in the vicious cycle of poverty, ignorance and deprivation. In this context, rabies is often not considered a high priority. A case needs to be built on DALYs lost, the economic losses resulting from rabies, and the benefits of effective rabies control in comparison with other diseases.

Training materials and course curricula for various categories of professional and support staff should be developed to increase awareness among medical health professionals of the importance and correct methods of wound cleansing, appropriate use of anti-rabies vaccines and utility of ERIG/HRIG. The need for special training is acute in peripheral areas where marketing of rabies biologicals and associated awareness by the private sector is also inadequate because of limited markets.

An important step in rabies control would be a situational analysis and reliable assessment of annual human and animal rabies deaths, animal bites, geographical distribution and other epidemiological information and data. In many countries, estimates of human rabies deaths are unchanged and have remained static for more than 10–15 years and no attempt is made at national level to collect accurate data and update or revise the figures. Countries should collect baseline data through appropriate surveys and should build strong epidemiological surveillance mechanisms.

12.2.5 *Availability of adequate quantities of modern immunizing agents for pre- and post-exposure treatment*

Many developing countries continue to produce and provide nerve-tissue vaccines through public hospitals and rabies treatment centres to the poorest segment of the population. In the same countries, the benefit of the safe and more potent tissue-culture vaccines are a prerogative of the rich and affluent. The fact that intradermal administration of tissue-culture vaccines for post-exposure prophylaxis is cost effective and eventually cheaper than nerve-tissue vaccines should be highlighted and brought to the attention of policy-makers.

12.2.6 Dog population management and mass immunization

Effective control of rabies requires a sound and practical dog population management relating to domestic, community and ownerless dog populations. Countries should develop effective integrated dog population management and immunization programmes. There is evidence that sustained and effective immunization of 70% of dogs in a given area can result in breaking the transmission of rabies. Endemic countries should launch mass vaccination programmes reaching an appropriate number of animals each year and maintain that level of herd immunity over time until elimination is achieved. Studies of the basic parameters of dog populations (size, turnover, accessibility and ownership status) should be conducted in as many representative areas as possible (e.g. urban, periurban and rural) in each country.

12.2.7 Community awareness

This is one of the biggest deficiencies in rabies control. Community awareness of all aspects of rabies is generally lacking or limited, be it first aid or management of animal bites, pre- and post-exposure prophylaxis, responsible pet dog ownership, dog population management, laboratory diagnosis, etc.

Regarding the immediate measures to be carried out after a bite exposure, there is inadequate knowledge of the crucial need to wash wounds with soap and running water and apply antiseptics. Practices such as the application of chillies and other pastes on the wound are common. Knowledge of post-exposure prophylaxis and where vaccine is available is also limited. People may also contact local traditional healers for treatment, thus losing precious time and increasing the danger of infection and death. In addition, the full course of vaccine may not be taken because of financial constraints or other reasons. There is also a belief that bites by small puppies are not harmful or are less so. The lack of responsible ownership of community dogs is an important issue that is often overlooked.

12.2.8 Advocacy for rabies prevention and control at national level

— Policy-makers should be informed about the burden of rabies and the need for a systematic and sustained control programme, sufficient resource allocation and resource mobilization, and intersectoral coordination.
— Senior-level managers in health departments and veterinary services should identify and give necessary support to programme officers at provincial and district levels.
— Private medical practitioners should be trained regarding wound treatment, and immunization choices and schedules.
— Media, religious leaders, local community leaders and other influential groups should be mobilized to create awareness and promote community involvement in rabies control activities.

Acknowledgments

The Expert Consultation wishes to acknowledge the special contributions to the drafting of the background document made by the following individuals: Dr Angelika Banzhoff, Head, Clinical Research and Medical Affairs, Chiron Vaccines, Marburg, Germany; Dr Jacques Barrat, Chief, Epidemiological Surveillance Unit on Wild Fauna and Domestic Carnivores, Research Laboratory on Rabies and Pathology of Wild Animals, National Centre on Veterinary and Food Studies (AFSSA), Malzéville, France; Dr Ray Butcher, Consultant, World Society for the Protection of Animals, London, England; Dr Anil Dutta, Senior Director, Medical Affairs, Sanofi Pasteur International, Lyon, France; Dr John Edwards, Regional Coordinator OIE, Bangkok, Thailand; Dr P.A.L. Harischandra, Public Health Veterinary Services, Colombo, Sri Lanka; Dr Brad Jennings, Head of Rabies Franchise, Chiron Vaccines, Bangkok, Thailand; Dr Darryn Knobel, Sir Alexander Robertson Centre for Tropical Medicine, Royal School of Veterinary Studies, University of Edinburgh, Scotland; Mr John W. Krebs, Public Health Scientist, Epidemiology Section, Viral and Rickettsial Zoonoses Branch, National Center for Infectious Diseases, Centers for Disease Control and Prevention, Atlanta, Georgia, USA; Dr Jean Lang, Program Leader, Traveler Vaccines and Endemic Risks, Sanofi Pasteur, Lyon, France; Dr Derek Lobo, Regional Advisor, Vector Borne Disease Control and Regional Focal Point for Leprosy Elimination, WHO Regional Office for South-East Asia, New Delhi, India; Dr Claudius Malerczyk, Clinical Team Leader, Clinical Research and Medical Affairs, Chiron Vaccines, Marburg, Germany; Dr S. Abdul Rahman, Retired Dean, Veterinary College, Banglore and Secretary, Commonwealth Veterinary Association, Bangalore, India; Dr André Regnault, Area Export Manager, Virbac, Carros, France; Dr François Sandre, International Director Product Range, Traveler Vaccines and Endemic Risks, Sanofi Pasteur International, Lyon, France; Dr Carolin L. Schumacher, Associate Director, Rabies Control Programmes, Grandes Prophylaxies Global Enterprise, Merial Ltd, Lyon, France; Dr Cicilia Windiyaningsih, Head, Partnership Section of Zoonoses, Directorate General of Communicable Disease Control and Environmental Health, Ministry of Health, Jakarta, Indonesia; and Dr Jean-Antoine Zinsou, Medical Manager, Traveler Vaccines and Endemic Risks, Sanofi Pasteur International, Lyon, France.

Special thanks are due to Dr Delphine Mc Adams for coordinating work on preparation of the background document.

References

1. *WHO Expert Committee on Rabies. Eighth report.* Geneva, World Health Organization, 1992 (WHO Technical Report Series, No. 824).

2. **Cleaveland S et al.** Estimating human rabies mortality in the United Republic of Tanzania from dog bite injuries. *Bulletin of the World Health Organization*, 2002, 80:304–310.

3. **Knobel DL et al.** Re-evaluating the burden of rabies in Africa and Asia. *Bulletin of the World health Organization*, 2005, 83(5):360–368.

4. *Assessing the burden of rabies in India. WHO sponsored national multi-centric rabies survey 2003. Final report. August 2003.* Bangalore, Association for Prevention and Control of Rabies in India (APCRI), 2003.

5. **Aubert MF.** Costs and benefits of rabies control in wildlife in France. *Revue Scientifique et Technique (International Office of Epizootics)*, 1999, 18(2):533–543.

6. *IX REDIPIRA meeting of directors of national programs for rabies control in Latin America. Final report. Santa Cruz de las Sierra, Bolivia, October 7–9, 2002.* Washington, DC, Pan American Health Organization, 2003.

7. **Meslin FX, Kaplan MM, Koprowski H, eds.** *Laboratory techniques in rabies*, 4th ed. Geneva, World Health Organization, 1996.

8. **Tordo N et al.** Rhabdoviridae. In: Fauquet CM et al., eds, *Virus taxonomy, VIIIth Report of the International Committee on Taxonomy of Viruses.* London, Elsevier/Academic Press, 2004:623–644.

9. **Badrane H et al.** Evidence of two lyssavirus phylogroups with distinct pathogenicity and immunogenicity. *Journal of Virology*, 2001, 75:3268–3276.

10. **Nadin-Davis SA et al.** Lyssavirus P gene characterisation provides insights into the phylogeny of the genus and identifies structural similarities and diversity within the encoded phosphoprotein. *Virology*, 2002, 298:286–305.

11. **Botvinkin AD et al.** Novel lyssaviruses isolated from bats in Russia. *Emerging Infectious Diseases*, 2003, 9:1623–1625.

12. **Mitrabhakdi E et al.** Difference in neuropathogenetic mechanisms in human furious and paralytic rabies. *Journal of the Neurological Sciences* (in press).

13. **Rupprecht CE, Hemachudha T.** Rabies. In: Scheld M, Whitley RJ, Marra C, eds. *Infections of the central nervous system.* Philadelphia, Lippincott, Williams & Wilkins, 2004:243–259.

14. **Laothamatas J et al.** MR imaging in human rabies. *AJNR. American Journal of Neuroradiology*, 2003, 24:1102–1109.

15. *Transport of infectious substances.* Geneva, World Health Organization, 2004 (WHO/CDS/CSR/LYO/2004.9; http://www.who.int/csr/resources/publications/WHO_CDS_CSR_LYO_2004_9, accessed 31 March 2005).

16. **Hirose JA, Bourhy H, Sureau P.** Retro-orbital route for the collection of brain specimens for rabies diagnosis. *Veterinary Record*, 1991, 129:291–292.

17. **Tong TR et al.** Trucut needle biopsy through superior orbital fissure for the

diagnosis of rabies. *Lancet*, 1999, 354 (9196):2137–2138.

18. *Manual of diagnostic tests and vaccines for terrestrial animals*, 5th ed. Paris, World Organisation for Animal Health, 2004 (http://www.oie.int/eng/normes/mmanual/A_00044.htm, accessed 31 March 2005).

19. **Bourhy H et al.** Comparative field evaluation of the fluorescent-antibody test, virus isolation from tissue culture, and enzyme immunodiagnosis for rapid diagnosis of rabies. *Journal of Clinical Microbiology*, 1989, 27:519–523.

20. **Hemachudha T, Wacharapluesadee S.** Ante-mortem diagnosis of human rabies. *Clinical Infectious Diseases*, 2004, 39:1085–1086.

21. **Crepin P et al.** Intravitam diagnosis of human rabies by PCR using saliva and cerebrospinal fluid. *Journal of Clinical Microbiology*, 1998, 36:1117–1121.

22. **Jackson AC et al.** Management of rabies in humans. *Clinical Infectious Diseases*, 2003, 36:60–63.

23. Requirements for rabies vaccine for human use. In: *WHO Expert Committee on Biological Standardization. Thirty-first report.* Geneva, World Health Organization, 1981, Annex 2 (WHO Technical Report Series, No. 658).

24. *WHO Expert Committee on Biological Standardization. Thirty-ninth report.* Geneva, World Health Organization, 1987 (WHO Technical Report Series, No. 760).

25. Requirements for rabies vaccine for human use. In: *WHO Expert Committee on Biological Standardization. Forty-third report.* Geneva, World Health Organization, 1994, Annex 4 (WHO Technical Report Series, No. 840).

26. Requirements for rabies vaccine (inactivated) for human use produced in continuous cell lines. In: *WHO Expert Committee on Biological Standardization. Forty-third report.* Geneva, World Health Organization, 1994, Annex 5 (WHO Technical Report Series, No. 840).

27. Requirements for the use of animal cells as *in vitro* substrates for the production of biologicals. In: *WHO Expert Committee on Biological Standardization. Forty-seventh report.* Geneva, World Health Organization, 1998, Annex 1 (WHO Technical Report Series, No. 878).

28. Guidelines for national authorities on quality assurance for biological products. In: *WHO Expert Committee on Biological Standardization. Forty-second report.* Geneva, World Health Organization, 1992, Annex 2 (WHO Technical Report Series, No. 822).

29. Regulation and licensing of biological products in countries with newly developing regulatory authorities. In: *WHO Expert Committee on Biological Standardization. Forty-fifth report.* Geneva, World Health Organization, 1995, Annex 1 (WHO Technical Report Series, No. 858).

30. *Report. Discussion on WHO requirements for rabies vaccine for human use: potency assay, World Health Organization, Geneva, Switzerland, 20 May 2003.* Geneva, World Health Organization, 2003 (http://www.who.int/biologicals/publications/meetings/areas/vaccines/rabies/en/Rabies%20vaccine%20meeting%20Final%20May%202003.pdf, accessed 15 April 2005).

31. *Report. Discussion on WHO requirements for rabies vaccine for human use,*

World Health Organization, Geneva, Switzerland, 4–5 May 2004. Geneva, World Health Organization, 2004 (http://www.who.int/biologicals/publications/meetings/areas/vaccines/rabies/en/Rabies%20vaccine%20meeting%20Final%20May%202004.pdf, accessed 15 April 2005).

32. *WHO Expert Committee on Rabies. Seventh report.* Geneva, World Health Organization, 1984 (WHO Technical Report Series, No. 709).

33. Guidelines for clinical evaluation of vaccines: regulatory expectations. In: *WHO Expert Committee on Biological Standardization. Fifty-second report.* Geneva, World Health Organization, 2004, Annex 1 (WHO Technical Report Series No. 924).

34. Guidelines for nonclinical evaluation of vaccines. In: *WHO Expert Committee on Biological Standardization. Fifty-fourth report.* Geneva, World Health Organization (WHO Technical Report Series, in press) (http://www.who.int/biologicals/publications/en/nonclinical_evaluation_vaccines_nov_2003.pdf).

35. *WHO recommendations on rabies post-exposure treatment and the correct technique of intradermal immunization against rabies.* Geneva, World Health Organization, 1997 (WHO/EMC/ZOO/96.6).

36. *Report of a WHO Consultation on Intradermal Application of Human Rabies Vaccines, Geneva, Switzerland, 13–14 March 1995.* Geneva, World Health Organization, 1995 (WHO/Rab.Res./95.47).

37. *Report of informal discussions on intradermal application of modern rabies vaccines for human post-exposure treatment, Geneva, Switzerland, 22 January 1993.* Geneva, World Health Organization, 1993 (WHO/Rab.Res./93.41).

38. **Dodet B, Meslin F-X, eds.** *Fourth international symposium on rabies control in Asia. Symposium proceedings, 5–9 March 2001, Hanoi, Viet Nam.* Montrouge, John Libbey Eurotext, 2001.

39. *Field application of oral rabies vaccines for dogs. Report of a WHO Consultation organized in collaboration with the Office International des Epizooties (OIE), Geneva, Switzerland, 20–22 July 1998.* Geneva, World Health Organization, 1998 (WHO/EMC/ZDI/98.15).

40. *Report of the Fifth Consultation on Oral Immunization of Dogs against Rabies. Organized by WHO with the participation of the Office International des Epizooties (OIE), Geneva, 20–22 June 1994.* Geneva, World Health Organization, 1994 (WHO/Rab.Res./94.45).

41. *Report of a WHO Consultation on Requirements and Criteria for Field Trials on Oral Rabies Vaccination of Dogs and Wild Carnivores, Geneva, 1–2 March 1989.* Geneva, World Health Organization, 1989 (WHO/Rab.Res./89.32).

42. *Report of the Fourth WHO Consultation on Oral Immunization of Dogs against Rabies, Geneva, 14–15 June 1993.* Geneva, World Health Organization, 1993 (WHO/Rab.Res./93.42).

43. **Vaughn JB, Gerhardt P, Peterson JCD.** Excretion of street rabies virus in saliva of cats. *JAMA: the Journal of the American Medical Association*, 1963, 184:705–708.

44. **Vaughn JB, Newell KW.** Excretion of street virus in saliva of dogs. *JAMA:*

the Journal of the American Medical Association, 1965, 193:363–368.

45. WHO strategies for the control and elimination of rabies in Asia. Report of a WHO interregional consultation. Geneva, Switzerland, 17–21 July 2001. Geneva, World Health Organization, 2002 (WHO/CDS/CSR/EPH/2002.8).

46. Matter HC et al. Study of the dog population and the rabies control activities in the Mirigama area of Sri Lanka. Acta Tropica, 2000, 75(1):95–108.

47. Guidelines for dog population management. Geneva, World Health Organization/World Society for the Protection of Animals, May 1990 (WHO/ZOON/90.165).

48. King AA et al., eds. Historical perspectives of rabies in Europe and the Mediterranean Basin. Paris, World Organisation for Animal Health, 2004.

49. Report of WHO/APHIS Consultation on Baits and Baiting Delivery Systems for Oral Immunization of Wildlife against Rabies. Colorado State University, Fort Collins, Colorado, 10–12 July 1990. Geneva, World Health Organization, 1990 (WHO/Rab. Res./90.36).

50. The oral vaccination of foxes against rabies. Report of the Scientific Committee on Animal Health and Animal Wildlife. Adopted on 23 October 2002. European Commission (http://europa.eu.int/comm/food/fs/sc/scah/outcome_en.html, accessed 15 April 2005).

51. Terrestrial animal health code, 11th ed. Paris, World Organisation for Animal Health, 2004, Part 2, Chapter 2.2.5 (http://www.oie.int/eng/normes/mcode/en_chapitre_2.2.5.htm, accessed 31 March 2005).

52. Briggs DJ et al. A comparison of two serological methods for detecting the immune response after rabies vaccination in dogs and cats being exported to rabies-free areas. Biologicals, 1998, 26(4):347–355.

53. Cliquet F, Aubert M, Sagné L. Development of a fluorescent antibody virus neutralisation test (FAVN) for the quantitation of rabies-neutralising antibody. Journal of Immunological Methods, 1998, 212:79–87.

54. King A, ed. Rabies in eastern and southern Africa — a seminar organized by the Central Veterinary Research Institute, Lusaka, cosponsored by FAO, WHO and OIE, Lusaka, Zambia, 2–5 June 1992. Lyon, Fondation Marcel Mérieux, 1992 (available at http://www.who.int/rabies/international_symposia).

55. Proceedings of the Southern and Eastern Rabies Group international symposium. Pietermartzburg, South African Republic, 29–30 April 1993 (available at http://www.who.int/rabies/international_symposia).

56. Bingham J, Bishop GC, King and A, eds. Proceedings of the third international conference of the Southern and Eastern African Rabies Group. Harare, Zimbabwe, 7–9 March 1995. Lyon, Fondation Marcel Mérieux, 1996 (available at http://www.who.int/rabies/international_symposia).

57. Kitala P et al., eds. Proceeding of the Southern and Eastern African Rabies Group Meeting, Nairobi, Kenya, 4–6 March 1997. Lyon, Fondation Marcel Mérieux, 1998 (available at http://www.who.int/rabies/international_symposia).

58. Rutebarika C et al., eds. Proceedings of the Southern and Eastern African Rabies Group/World Health Organization meeting, Entebbe, Uganda, 29–31

March 1999. Lyon, Fondation Marcel Mérieux, 2000 (available at http://www.who.int/rabies/international_symposia).

59. **King A, Barrat J, eds.** *Proceedings of the Southern and Eastern African Rabies Group/World Health Organization meeting, Lilongwe, Malawi, 18–22 June 2001* (available at http://www.who.int/rabies/international_symposia).

60. **Barrat J, Nel L, eds.** *Proceedings of the Southern and Eastern African Rabies Group/World Health Organization meeting, Ezulwini, Swaziland, 12–15 May 2003* (available at http://www.who.int/rabies/international_symposia).

61. *Report of the workshop on rabies control in Asian countries. Samarkand, September 19–21, 1989.* Lyon, Fondation Marcel Mérieux, 1990.

62. *Proceedings of the symposium on rabies control in Asia. Jakarta, Indonesia, 27–30 April 27–30, 1993.* Lyon, Fondation Marcel Mérieux, 1994.

63. **Dodet B, Meslin FX, eds.** *Rabies control in Asia. Third international symposium on rabies control in Asia. 11–15 September 1996, Wuhan, China.* Paris, Elsevier, 1997.

64. *WHO meeting of rabies control in middle and east European Countries, in Kosice Slovakia, September 25th–27th 2002* (organized by the WHO Collaborating Centre for Rabies Surveillance and Research). Insel Riems, Friedrich Loeffler Institute (http://www.fli.bund.de/).

65. **Bahloul C et al.** Perrin DNA-based immunisation for exploring the enlargement of immunological cross-reactivity against the lyssaviruses. *Vaccine*, 1998, 16:417–425.

66. **Jallet C et al.** Chimeric lyssavirus glycoproteins with increased immunological potential. *Journal of Virology*, 1999, 73:225–233.

67. **Desmezières E et al.** Lyssavirus glycoproteins expressing immunologically potent B cell and cytotoxic T lymphocyte epitopes as prototypes for multivalent vaccines. *Journal of General Virology*, 1999, 80:2343–2351.

Annex 1
Guide for post-exposure prophylaxis

A1. General considerations

The recommendations given here are intended as a general guide. It is understood that, in certain situations, modifications of these recommendations may be warranted. Such situations include, but are not limited to: exposure of infants or mentally disabled people to a suspect or confirmed rabid animal; and when a reliable exposure history cannot be ascertained, particularly in areas where rabies is enzootic, even when the animal is considered to be healthy at the time of exposure. A careful risk assessment should be conducted by a qualified medical professional on every patient exposed to a potentially rabid animal (see section 6.2).

Post-exposure prophylaxis consists of local treatment of the wound, initiated as soon as possible after an exposure, followed by the administration of passive immunization, if indicated, and a potent and effective rabies vaccine that meets WHO criteria (see section 5). Post-exposure prophylaxis may be discontinued if the animal involved is a dog or cat that remains healthy for an observation period of 10 days after the exposure occurred; or if the animal is humanely killed and proven to be negative for rabies by a reliable diagnostic laboratory using a prescribed test. If the animal inflicting the wound is suspected of being rabid and is not apprehended, post-exposure prophylaxis should be instituted immediately. When animal bites occur in a rabies-free area where adequate rabies surveillance is in effect, post-exposure prophylaxis may not be required depending upon the outcome of a risk assessment conducted by a medical expert knowledgeable in the epidemiology of rabies in the area and the proper requirements for assessing the risk involved (see section 6.2). In areas where canine or wildlife rabies is enzootic, adequate laboratory surveillance is in place, and data from laboratory and field experience indicate that there is no infection in the species involved, local health authorities may not recommend anti-rabies prophylaxis.

A2. Local treatment of wounds

Elimination of rabies virus at the site of the infection by chemical or physical means is an effective mechanism of protection. Therefore, the Consultation emphasized the importance of prompt local treatment of all bite wounds and scratches that might be contaminated with rabies virus. Recommended first-aid procedures include immediate and thorough flushing and washing of the wound for a minimum of 15 minutes with soap and water, detergent, povidone iodine or other substances of proven lethal effect on rabies virus. If soap or an antiviral agent is not available, the wound should be thoroughly and extensively washed with water. People who live in rabies-infected areas should be educated in simple local wound treatment and warned not to use procedures that may further contaminate the wounds. Most severe bite wounds are best treated by daily dressing followed by secondary suturing where necessary. If suturing after wound cleansing cannot be avoided, the wound should first be infiltrated with passive rabies immunization products and suturing delayed for several hours. This will allow diffusion of the antibody to occur through the tissues before suturing is performed. Other treatments, such as the administration of antibiotics and tetanus prophylaxis, should be applied as appropriate for other bite wounds.

A3. Administration of rabies biologicals for passive immunization

The role of passive rabies immunization products is to provide the immediate availability of neutralizing antibodies at the site of the exposure before it is physiologically possible for the patient to begin producing his or her own antibodies after vaccination. Therefore, passive immunization products should be administered to all patients presenting with exposure to rabies-infected material onto mucous membranes or into transdermal wounds.

A3.1 *Classes of rabies biologicals and precautions for their use*

There are three classes of rabies biological products for passive immunization available at present: human rabies immunoglobulin (HRIG); equine rabies immunoglobulin (ERIG), and highly purified F(ab')2 products produced from ERIG. Most ERIG products currently being manufactured are highly purified and the occurrence of adverse events has been significantly reduced. Given that the clearance of F(ab')2 fragments is more rapid than intact immunoglobulins, the Consultation recommended that in cases of multiple severe exposures, HRIG should be used for passive immunization. Most of the new ERIG preparations are potent, highly purified, safe and considerably less expensive than HRIG. However, they are of heterologous origin and carry a small risk of hypersensitivity reactions and therefore a skin test should be conducted prior to administration of ERIG and F(ab')2 products according to the guidelines of the manufacturer. Serum sickness, using a highly purified ERIG product, appears among <1–2% of recipients and usually develops 1 week after administration. In the event of a positive skin test to ERIG or a F(ab')2 product, HRIG should be administered. If HRIG is not available, ERIG or F(ab')2 products should still be used but should be administered under the close supervision of competent staff located in adequate medical facilities.

A3.2 *Dosage and administration*

The dose for HRIG is 20 IU/kg body weight, and for ERIG and F(ab')2 products is 40 IU/kg body weight. As much of the recommended dose of passive immunization products as is anatomically feasible should be infiltrated into and around the wounds. Multiple needle injections into the wound should be avoided. If a finger or toe needs to be infiltrated, care must be taken not to cause a compartment syndrome, which can occur when an excessive volume is infiltrated under pressure and blood circulation is impaired. In the event that a remainder of passive rabies immunization product is left after all wounds have been infiltrated, it should be administered by deep intramuscular injection at an injection site distant from the vaccine injection site. Animal bite wounds inflicted can be severe and multiple, especially in small children. In such cases, the calculated dose of the passive rabies immunization product may not be sufficient to infiltrate all wounds. In these circumstances, it is advisable to dilute the passive immunization product in normal saline to a sufficient volume to be able to inject all wounds. A full course of vaccine should follow thorough wound cleansing and passive immunization.

A4. Vaccine administration for active immunization

Intramuscular regimens
Cell-culture or purified embryonated egg rabies vaccines having a potency of at least 2.5 IU per single intramuscular immunizing dose should be applied according to one of the following regimens.

— Five-dose intramuscular regimen (Essen regimen)

One dose of vaccine is administered intramuscularly on days 0, 3, 7, 14 and 28. Injections must be given in the upper arm (deltoid region) or, in small children, into the anterolateral thigh muscle. *Vaccine should never be administered into the gluteal region, where absorption is unpredictable.*

— Abbreviated multisite intramuscular regimen ("2–1–1" or Zagreb regimen)

One dose of vaccine is administered intramuscularly into the left and one into the right upper arm (deltoid region) on day 0 followed by one dose into the upper arm (deltoid region) on days 7 and 21. This schedule saves two clinic visits and one vaccine dose.

Intradermal regimens

A limited number of rabies vaccines has been recognized to date by WHO as safe and efficacious for post-exposure prophylaxis when administered by the intradermal route in two different regimens. Local manufacturers in rabies-endemic countries are beginning to produce rabies vaccines. The intradermal use of these vaccines should be based on adherence to WHO requirements for that route and approval by national health authorities (see section 5). New vaccine manufacturers should provide clinical evidence that their products are immunogenic and safe when used intradermally. Clinical evidence should include clinical trials involving a vaccine of known immunogenicity and efficacy when used by this route as control, serological testing with rapid fluorescent focus inhibition test, and publication in internationally peer-reviewed journals.

— Updated Thai Red Cross intradermal regimen ("2–2–2–0–2" regimen)

Sufficient clinical evidence was presented to the Consultation indicating that a single dose of vaccine given on day 90 of the original Thai Red Cross regimen ("2–2–2–0–1–1" regimen) can be replaced if two doses of vaccine are given on day 28 ("2–2–2–0–2" regimen). The Thai Red Cross regimen considerably lowers the cost of vaccination as the total volume of vaccine required is much less than that needed for intramuscular regimens.

The schedule for the updated Thai Red Cross intradermal regimen is as follows: one dose of vaccine, in a volume of 0.1 ml is given intradermally at two different lymphatic drainage sites, usually the left and right upper arm, on days 0, 3, 7 and 28. Vaccine administered intradermally must raise a visible and palpable "bleb" in the skin. In the event that a dose of vaccine is inadvertently given subcutaneously or intramuscularly, a new dose should be administered intradermally. Currently there are two vaccines that have been proven to be efficacious in the Thai Red Cross regimen: purified Vero cell rabies vaccine produced by Aventis Pasteur and purified chick embryo cell rabies vaccine produced by Chiron Vaccines.

— Eight-site intradermal regimen ("8–0–4–0–1–1" regimen)

One dose of 0.1 ml is administered intradermally at eight different sites (upper arms, lateral thighs, suprascapular region, and lower quadrant of abdomen) on day 0. On day 7, four 0.1 ml injections are administered intradermally into each upper arm (deltoid region) and each lateral thigh. Following these injections, one additional 0.1 ml dose is administered on days 28 and 90. This regimen lowers the cost of vaccine administered by intramuscular regimens and generally produces a higher antibody response than the other recommended schedules by day 14. It does not result in a significantly earlier antibody response and in order to ensure optimal treatment, a passive immune product must be administered to patients presenting with severe exposures. Only two commercial products are today considered safe and efficacious when administered according to this regimen. They include a human diploid cell vaccine produced by Aventis Pasteur and a purified chick embryo cell rabies vaccine produced by Chiron Vaccines.

Intradermal injections must be administered by staff trained in this technique. Vaccine vials should be stored between 2 °C and 8 °C after reconstitution and the total content should be used as soon as possible, but at least within 8 hours. Rabies vaccines formulated with an adjuvant should not be administered intradermally.

A5. Post-exposure prophylaxis of previously vaccinated people

Individuals who are not immunocompromised and who have been previously vaccinated with a potent and effective rabies vaccine that meets WHO criteria for vaccine production and have adequate documentation should receive a two-booster series consisting of one intramuscular or intradermal dose on days 0 and 3. The administration of passive immunization is not required.

Local wound treatment should be completed as noted above. People who have received pre-exposure or post-exposure vaccination using a vaccine of unproven potency, should receive a full post-exposure vaccination series including passive immunization.

A6. Post-exposure prophylaxis of HIV-infected people and HIV/AIDS patients

Several studies of patients with HIV/AIDS have reported that those with very low CD4 counts will mount a significantly lower or no detectable neutralizing antibody response to rabies. In such patients and those in whom the presence of immunological memory is no longer assured as a result of other causes, proper and thorough wound treatment as described above and antisepsis accompanied by local infiltration of a passive immunization product are of utmost importance.

Immunocompromised patients with category II exposures should receive rabies immunoglobulin in addition to a full post-exposure vaccination series as listed above. An infectious disease specialist with expert knowledge of rabies prevention should be consulted.

A7. Type of contact, exposure and recommended post-exposure prophylaxis

Table A1 should serve as a guide for post-exposure prophylaxis. In cases where exposure is questionable or a patient has a concurrent medical condition that may complicate post-exposure prophylaxis, an expert in the administration of rabies prophylaxis should be consulted.

Table A1

Type of contact, exposure and recommended post-exposure prophylaxis

Category	Type of contact with a suspect or confirmed rabid domestic or wild[a] animal, or animal unavailable for testing	Type of exposure	Recommended post-exposure prophylaxis
I	Touching or feeding of animals Licks on intact skin	None	None, if reliable case history is available
II	Nibbling of uncovered skin Minor scratches or abrasions without bleeding	Minor	Administer vaccine immediately[b] Stop treatment if animal remains healthy throughout an observation period of 10 days[c] or if animal is proven to be negative for rabies by a reliable laboratory using appropriate diagnostic techniques
III	Single or multiple transdermal bites or scratches, licks on broken skin Contamination of mucous membrane with saliva (i.e. licks) Exposures to bats[d]	Severe	Administer rabies immunoglobulin and vaccine immediately. Stop treatment is animal remains healthy throughout an observation period of 10 days or if animal is found to be negative for rabies by a reliable laboratory using appropriate diagnostic techniques

[a] Exposure to rodents, rabbits and hares seldom, if ever, requires specific anti-rabies post-exposure prophylaxis.
[b] If an apparently healthy dog or cat in or from a low-risk area is placed under observation, the situation may warrant delaying initiation of treatment.
[c] This observation period applies only to dogs and cats. Except in the case of threatened or endangered species, other domestic and wild animals suspected as rabid should be humanely killed and their tissues examined for the presence of rabies antigen using appropriate laboratory techniques.
[d] Post-exposure prophylaxis should be considered when contact between a human and a bat has occurred unless the exposed person can rule out a bite or scratch, or exposure to a mucous membrane.

Annex 2
Suggested rabies vaccination certificate for humans

The vaccination certificate below is provided as a model for copying. It should be kept carefully by the vaccinee with his or her personal health documents. Blank forms should be supplied by the manufacturer of the vaccine.

RABIES VACCINATION CERTIFICATE

Name _____

Date of birth _____ Sex _____

Signature _____

Address _____

_____ Tel. no. _____

PRE-EXPOSURE VACCINATION

Primary vaccination:

Date	Dose/route/site of administration	Type of vaccine (origin/batch no.)	Vaccination center of physician	Signature
_____	_____	_____	_____	_____
_____	_____	_____	_____	_____
_____	_____	_____	_____	_____

Serum titre, if determined: _____

Booster:

Date	Dose/route/site of administration	Type of vaccine (origin/batch no.)	Vaccination center	Signature of physician
_____	_____	_____	_____	_____
_____	_____	_____	_____	_____
_____	_____	_____	_____	_____

POST-EXPOSURE PROPHYLAXIS

1. Rabies immunoglobulin (human or equine origin):

Date   Dose (IU)   Origin

_____   _____   _____

2. Vaccine:

Date	Dose/route/site of administration	Type of vaccine (origin/batch no.)	Vaccination center	Signature of physician
_____	_____	_____	_____	_____
_____	_____	_____	_____	_____
_____	_____	_____	_____	_____

3. Category of contact: _____

Annex 3
Addresses of international institutions for technical cooperation in rabies control

The following WHO collaborating centres and other international organizations and institutions are prepared to collaborate with national services on request.

Collaborating and related reference centres for rabies

The Director
WHO Collaborating Centre for Control,
Pathogenesis and Epidemiology
of Rabies in Carnivores
Centre of Expertise (COFE) for Rabies
Ottawa Laboratory Fallowfield (OLF)
Canadian Food Inspection Agency
3851 Fallowfield Road, P.O. Box 11300
Station H, Nepean, K2H 8P9
Ontario
Canada

Tel.: +1 613 228 6698
Fax: +1 613 228 6669

The Director
WHO Collaborating Centre for the
Rabies inCharacterization of Rabies
and Rabies-related Viruses
Department of Virology
Veterinary Laboratories Agency
New Haw, Addlestone
Weybridge, Surrey, KT15 3NB
England

Tel.: +44 1932-357840
Fax: +44 1932-357239
http://www.defra.gov.uk/
corporate/via

The Director
WHO Collaborating Centre for
Research and Management on
Zoonoses Control
Research Laboratory on Rabies and
Pathology of Wild Animals
National Centre on Veterinary and Food
Studies (AFSSA)
Domaine de Pixérécourt, B.P. 9
F-54220 Malzéville
France

Tel.: +33 3 83 29 89 50
Fax: +33 3 83 29 89 59

The Director WHO Collaborating Centre for Reference and Research on Rabies Pasteur Institute rue du Docteur Roux F-75724 Paris Cedex 15 France	Tel.: +33 1 45 68 87 50 Fax: +33 1 40 61 30 20 http://www.pasteur.fr
The Director WHO Collaborating Centre for Rabies Surveillance and Research Institute of Epidemiology Federal Research Centre for Animal Virus Diseases Seestrasse 55 D-16868 Wusterhausen Germany	Tel.: +49 33979 80816 Fax. +49 33979 80200 http://www.bfav.de
The Director WHO Collaborating Centre for Reference and Research in Rabies Department of Neurovirology National Institute of Mental Health and Neurosciences (NIMHANS) Hosur Road Bangalore 560029 India	Tel.: +91 80 699 5128/9 Fax: +91 80 6562121
The Director WHO Collaborating Centre for Rabies Epidemiology National Institute of Communicable Diseases (NICD) 22 Sham Nath Marg Post Box 1492 New Delhi 110 054 India	Tel.: +9111 252 1272/252 1524 Fax: +9111 233 482
The Director WHO Collaborating Centre for Reference and Research on Rabies Pasteur Institute of Iran 69 Pasteur Avenue 13164 Tehran Islamic Republic of Iran	Tel.: +9821 640 3496 Fax: +9821 646 5132 http://www.pasteur.ac.ir

The Director
WHO Collaborating Centre for
Research on Rabies Pathogenesis
and Prevention
Queen Saovabha Memorial Institute
Thai Red Cross Society
Rama IV Road
10330 Bangkok
Thailand

Tel.: +66 2 252 6117
Fax: +66 2 254 0212

The Director
WHO Collaborating Centre for
Reference and Research on Rabies
Rabies Section
Center for Infectious Diseases
Centers for Diseases Control
1600 Clifton Road, Atlanta, GA 30333
USA

Tel: +1 404 639 1050
Fax: +1 404 639 3163
http://www.cdc.gov

The Director
WHO Collaborating Centre for
Reference and Research on Rabies
The Wistar Institute
3601 Spruce Street
Philadelphia, PA 19104-4268
USA

Tel.: +1 215 898 3863
Fax: +1 215 898 3953
http://www.wistar.upenn.edu

The Director
WHO Collaborating Centre for
Neurovirology
Department of Immunology and
Microbiology
Thomas Jefferson University
1020 Locus Street
Philadelphia, PA 19107–6799
USA

Tel.: +1 215 503 4761
Fax: +1 215 923 6795
http://www.greenvaccines.org

WHO regional offices

Regional Director
WHO Regional Office for Africa
Bureau Annexe
P.O. Box BE 773
Harare
Zimbabwe

Tel.: +47 241 38066
Fax: +263 4 746 823/127
http://www.afro.who.int

Regional Director
WHO Regional Office for the Americas/
Pan American Sanitary Bureau
525, 23rd Street NW
Washington, DC 20037
USA

Tel.: +1 202 861 3200
Fax: +1 202 223 5971
http://www.paho.org

Regional Director
WHO Regional Office for the Eastern
Mediterranean
P.O. Box 7608
Cairo 11371
Egypt

Tel.: +20 2 2765280
Fax: +20 2 2765414
http://www.emro.who.int

Regional Director
WHO Regional Office for Europe
8 Scherfigsvej
DK2100 Copenhagen
Denmark

Tel.: +45 39 17 13 98
Fax: +45 39 17 18 51
http://www.euro.who.int

Regional Director
WHO Regional Office for South-East
Asia
World Health House
Indraprastha Estate
Mahatma Gandhi Road
New Delhi 110 002
India

Tel.: +91 11 23370804
Fax: +91 11 23378412
http://www.whosea.org

Regional Director
WHO Regional Office for the Western
Pacific
P.O. Box 2932
Manila 1100
Philippines

Tel.: +63 2 528 8001
Fax: +63 2 521 1036
http://www.wpro.who.int

Other international organizations

Director
Animal Production and Health Division
Food and Agriculture Organization of
the United Nations (FAO)
Via delle Terme di Caracalla
I-00100 Rome
Italy

Tel.: +39 06 570 54102
Fax: +39 06 570 53152
http://www.fao.org/UNFAO

Director-General
World Organisation for Animal Health
(OIE)
12 rue de Prony
F-75017 Paris
France

Tel.: +33 1 44 15 18 88
Fax: +33 1 42 67 09 87
http://www.oie.int

Nongovernmental organizations

International Union for the of
Conservation Nature and Natural
Resources (IUCN)
Avenue du Mont-Blanc
1196 Gland
Switzerland

Tel.: +41 22 649 114
Fax: +41 22 642 926
http://www.iucn.org

World Society for the Protection of
Animals (WSPA)
89 Albert Embankment
London SE1 7TP
England

Tel.: +44 20 7587 5000
Fax: +44 20 7793 0208
http://www.wspa.org.uk

Marwar Trust
12 Rue François Bonivard
1201 Geneva
Switzerland

Tel.: +41 22 716 0035
Fax: +41 22 716 0002
http://www.marwartrust.org

Annex 4
International rabies vaccination certificate for dogs, cats and ferrets

The vaccination certificate below is provided as a model for copying.

CERTIFICAT INTERNATIONAL DE VACCINATION ANTIRABIQUE POUR CHIENS, CHATS ET FURETS/INTERNATIONAL RABIES VACCINATION CERTIFICATE FOR DOGS, CATS AND FERRETS

I. Propriétaire/Owner

Nom et adresse
Name and address _____

_____

_____

II. Signalement/Description

Espèce
Species _____

Age ou date de naissance (si possible)
Age or date of birth (where known) _____

Sexe
Sex _____

Race
Breed _____

Robe
Coat colour _____

Type de pelage et marques/signes particuliers
Coat type and marking/distinguishing marks _____

Numéro de micro chip
Microchip no. _____

Type de lecteur du micro chip
Microchip scanner type _____

Emplacement du micro chip
Location of microchip _____

Numéro et emplacement du tatouage (si présent)
Location and tattoo no. (if applicable) _____

III. Vaccinations antirabiques/Rabies vaccinations

Le soussigné certifie avoir vacciné contre la rage l'animal décrit à la page 1, comme il est indiqué ci-après. Au moment de la vaccination, l'animal a été reconnu en bonne santé.

The undersigned declares herewith that she or he has vaccinated the animal described on page 1 against rabies, as shown below. The animal was found to be health.

(1) Date de vaccination Vaccination date	(2) Valable jusqu'au Valid until	(3) Nom du vaccin Name of vaccine	(4) Nom du fabricant Name of manufacturer	(5) Numéro de lot Batch no.	(6) signature et cachet du vétérinaire officiel Signature and stamp of official veterinary surgeon

IV. Tests sérologiques antirabiques/Rabies serological tests

Déclaration du vétérinaire/Veterinary declaration

Je soussigné(e) certifie avoir pris connaissance des résultats officiels du test sérologique pratiqué sur l'animal décrit ci-dessus à la date du (jj/mm/aa)_____, conduit par un laboratoire agréé confirmant que le titre d'anticorps neutralisants anti-rage était supérieur ou égal à 0.5 UI/ml.

Nom, date, et cachet du vétérinaire officiel

I have seen an official record of the result of a serological test for the animal, carried out on a sample taken on (dd/mm/yy) _____ and tested in an approved laboratory, which states that the rabies-neutralizing antibody titre was equal to or greater than 0.5 IU/ml.

Name, date and signature of the authorized veterinarian:

Tests supplémentaires/Further tests:

Date	Résultat Result	Laboratoire agréé Approved laboratory	Signature et cachet du vétérinaire Signature and stamp of veterinary surgeon

V. Autres vaccinations/Other vaccinations

Date	Vaccin utilisé Type of vaccine	Numéro de lot Batch no.	Signature et cachet du vétérinaire Signature and stamp of veterinary surgeon

VI. Informations complémentaires/Additional information

Pays d'origine/Country of origin

Pays dans lesquels l'animal a séjourné, selon les déclarations du propriétaire (indiquer les dates)/Countries visited by the animal as declared by the owner (give dates)

_____

_____

_____

_____

Notes

Le présent certificat ne dispense pas de l'application des autres dispositions en vigueur pour l'entrée dans chaque pays. Prière de lire la section VII.

This certificate may not be sufficient to meet all the requirements of the countries of destination. Please read Section VII.

Autorisation d'imprimer délivrée par (indiquer l'autorité national compétente):

Printing authorized by (indicate the national responsible authority):

_____

Pour être valable, le présent certificat doit porter un numéro perforé à chaque page.

To be valid, this certificate must bear a number perforated on each page.

VII. Passage de frontière/Frontier crossing

1. Le propriétaire de l'animal doit, avant de se rendre à l'étranger avec celui-ci, s'assurer des conditions sanitaires imposées par les autorités du pays de destination, le présent certificat ne dispensant pas de l'application des autres dispositions en vigueur dans certains pays.

   The owner of the animal must, before going abroad with it, make sure of the veterinary requirements laid down by the authorities of the country of destination, as this certificate may not be sufficient to meet all the requirements of the country of destination.

2. Le présent certificat est valable à partir du trentième jour et jusqu'à la fin du douzième mois après la date de la première vaccination; dans le cas d'une revaccination au cours de la période de validité, pendant les douze mois qui suivent la date de revaccination. This certificate is valid from the 30th day until the end of the 12th month after the date of the first vaccination; in the case of

revaccination within the validity period, for 12 months from the date of revaccination.

3. Le présent certificat doit être imprimé et complété en Français et en Anglais, et si nécessaire, dans la langue du pays d'origine.

This certificate must be printed and completed in French and English and, if necessary, the language of the country of origin.

Annex 5
Suggested case-record form for human exposure to rabies

The form below is provided as a model for copying.

SUGGESTED CASE-rECORD FORM
FOR HUMAN EXPOSURE TO RABIES

Case no._____   Referred by_____

Person bitten

Name_____   Date of bite _____

Age _____   Geographical locality of biting episode

                               _____

Home address _____   Site(s) of bite on the body_____

                               Nature of bite _____

Other persons (if any)   Single ☐   Mild   ☐

                               Multiple ☐   Moderate ☐

                                              Severe   ☐

Other persons (if any)   1._____

bitten by the same animal   2._____

(names and addresses)   3._____

                               4._____

Treatment

Local wound treatment _____

Vaccine: ### *Immunoglobulins:*

Type of vaccine (brain-derived or   Source of rabies immunoglobulin (RIG):

cell-culture)_____   Human ☐   Animal ☐

Manufacturer and batch no._____   Manufacturer and batch no. _____

_____   _____

Route of administration:_____   Dose administered _____

Size or quantity administered _____   Results of sensitivity test _____

Dates administered _____   Date administered_____

_____

_____

_____

Previous rabies vaccines administered?__   Previous RIG administered?_____

Date_____ Date_____

Type_____ Type_____

Were there undesirable effects following treatment? If yes, specify treatment, nature of side-effects and outcome _____

_____

Status of exposed person after 6 months:

Alive   ☐

Died of rabies   ☐   Date of death _____

Died of other causes   ☐

Unknown   ☐

Status of other persons bitten by the same animal, if known: _____

_____

Biting animal:

Animal species _____

Breed _____ Age_____

Sex _____ Weight _____

Was the animal vaccinated against rabies? _____

If yes, type of vaccine _____ Date _____

Outcome:

Under observation ☐   Killed ☐   Escaped ☐

Outcome after_____ days: _____ Results of laboratory tests:

Signs of rabies   ☐   positive negative

Healthy   ☐   Florescent antibody test ☐   ☐

Died   ☐   Negri bodies   ☐   ☐

                                Animal inoculation   ☐   ☐

                                Other tests   ☐   ☐

Annex 6
Rabnet, an interactive and information mapping system for human and animal rabies[1]

DATA QUERY

INTERACTIVE MAPS

MAPS & RESOURCES

Registered Users Login

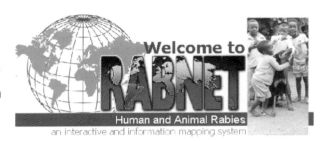

Since 1959, the World Health Organization has collected data on human and animal rabies from its Member States using the World Rabies Survey (WRS) questionnaire. In the late 1990s, a web-based electronic version of the questionnaire accessible through Rabnet was added to the paper version sent by surface or airmail. Over the past 2 years, rabies data collection and processing online have been improved. We are therefore proud to announce the release of "Rabnet version 2".

"Rabnet 2" provides new features such as the possibility to create interactive global or country rabies maps. In the near future it will be possible to generate rabies maps at district and even community level. "Rabnet 2" also has a library of ready-made maps and rabies-related documents and also provides details of the network of WHO collaborating centres for rabies. Finally, in "Rabnet 2" rabies data can be linked to a broad range of country-specific indicators (population, education and health services) to provide a more comprehensive picture of the situation in various geographical areas.

With this new system the "**data questionnaire**" can be accessed and data entered online. Main rabies indicators have been reviewed and the number of questions has been consequently reduced. Once validated, data are automatically transferred into the "Rabnet 2" for your immediate access and processing.

A username and password are required to get access to the online questionnaire. Access to the Rabnet data bank and other features is freely available.

For further information, please contact: rabnet@who.int

---

[1] http://www.who.int/rabies/rabnet